Management of the
Addicted Patient in Primary Care

T0235652

Management of the Addicted Patient in Primary Care

Heidi Allespach Pomm, PhD
Faculty and Coordinator of Behavioral Science, Family Medicine Residency Program, St. Vincent's Medical Center, Jacksonville, Florida; Clinical Associate Professor, College of Osteopathic Medicine, Nova Southeastern University, Ft. Lauderdale, Florida; Voluntary Faculty, Department of Family Medicine and Community Health, University of Miami Miller School of Medicine, Miami, Florida

Raymond M. Pomm, MD
Medical Director, Florida Impaired Practitioners Program; Medical Director, River Region Human Services; Medical Director, Gateway Community Services; Expert Consultant to the Florida Board of Bar Examiners in Matters Related to Impairment; Clinical Assistant Professor, Department of Psychiatry, University of Florida, Gainesville, Florida

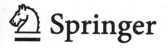 Springer

Heidi Allespach Pomm, PhD
Faculty and Coordinator of Behavioral Science, Family Medicine Residency Program, St. Vincent's Medical Center, Jacksonville, Florida; Clinical Associate Professor, College of Osteopathic Medicine, Nova Southeastern University, Ft. Lauderdale, Florida; Voluntary Faculty, Department of Family Medicine and Community Health, University of Miami Miller School of Medicine, Miami, Florida

Raymond M. Pomm, MD
Medical Director, Florida Impaired Practitioners Program; Medical Director, River Region Human Services; Medical Director, Gateway Community Services; Expert Consultant to the Florida Board of Bar Examiners in Matters Related to Impairment; Clinical Assistant Professor, Department of Psychiatry, University of Florida, Gainesville, Florida

Library of Congress Control Number: 2007921868

ISBN 978-0-387-35961-8   ISBN 978-0-387-71885-9 (eBook)

Printed on acid-free paper.

I dedicate this book to my father and exemplary psychiatrist, Dr. Bruce Walter Alspach, and to my wonderful mother, Mrs. Maxine Farr Alspach, for their unwavering, unconditional love and support throughout the years. No one could ever ask for better parents than you.

I also dedicate this book to my dear and beloved friend, Dianne Gars. Thank you for sharing your "experience, strength, and hope" and for always standing strong beside me during all of these years. I am so grateful you were put into my life, and I love you more than words can ever express.

To the millions of recovering alcoholics and addicts who have had the courage to move from the darkness of active disease into the light of sobriety . . . thank you for all you have taught me, and may your lives always be "happy, joyous, and free!"

Last but never least, this book is dedicated with a tremendous amount of love and admiration to my "team"; my amazing, smart, beautiful, and incredibly big-hearted daughter, Summer; and my wonderful husband and soulmate, Ray. I cherish the love you both give me more than anything in the world, and this book would not have been possible without you.

—HP

I dedicate this book to my family. First, to my parents, Monty and Eileen, who, beyond raising me, were there in so many ways as I traveled this tortuous journey through life. Their expectations and modeling steered my academic and professional direction. Their support has been consistent and backed by a lifetime of love.

My sister, Laureen: whose life's decisions started me on my journey into the field of psychiatry. Even though she has lived in a foreign country, her presence and unconditional love have always been felt.

My son, David, has loved me and, with wisdom beyond his years, understood my busy work schedule. His acceptance and respect have been realized at my core, fueling my desire to be the very best I can be for him and for all those around me.

My new daughter, Summer, has showered me with a love I would never have experienced. Her presence in my life has brought a new light to help brighten the way. She has shown me a new energy that has strengthened my belief in the future, for both those who are healthy and those who are ill.

Last, but certainly not least, my wife, Heidi: my best friend, my life partner, my lover, and my soulmate. She has always been by my side, forever supporting me, even when life seems so overwhelming. Without her, this book would never have been written. She is the love of my life.

—RP

Foreword

Tobacco, alcohol, illicit drugs, and secondhand exposure are the nation's leading health problems. These acquired problems cause more than half of all deaths per year. First use, as well as some subsequent use, may be voluntary, but after loss of control, continued use is to be expected in an addict. So, prevention is the treatment of choice and also the treatment with the greatest efficacy. When prevention fails, early intervention and prompt treatment are critical; otherwise, abuse becomes dependence and with it comes a chronic life-long disease without a specific cure. This places a great deal of responsibility on the already overburdened primary care physicians, who must identify a disease fraught with denial and whose patients are generally the last ones to know and accept the fact that they are hopelessly addicted and need help. Physician education and competency make early diagnosis more likely, but most practicing physicians do not have addiction education or treatment training as part of their undergraduate medical education. Among physicians, tobacco competency has improved, and a smoking history is now a part of almost every new patient assessment. A patient's attempts to quit and pharmacologic treatments have been incorporated into most practices in which the physician emphasizes wellness. Most physicians have prescribed and followed patients treated with nicotine replacement and Zyban. Progress in the treatment of alcohol abuse and dependence, cocaine and prescription misuse and dependence, and other drugs of abuse has been much slower.

All drugs of abuse have similar net effects on the brain and cause a substance abuse dependence syndrome that is stereotyped and consistent whether the patient is homeless or a physician. Our group has worked to understand the likely neurobiology of addictions. Our work and the work of others, such as Koob and Volkow, with opioid drugs and the noradrenergic systems, cocaine and the dopamine systems, and tobacco and cannabinoids has been well referenced and summarized where appropriate. Like ourselves, Pomm and Pomm understand that detoxification, whether fast or slower or whether with this medication or that, is rarely a treatment. Detoxification is a first step in the treatment of dependence, but treatment really begins after detox. Although cutting-edge science has a central place in this text, the focus is clearly not on science for science's sake, but rather on the research that translates to people. It is one thing to point out that the brain has cannabinoid receptors and that they have a certain distribution and evolutionary biology. It is quite another to point out that these systems can be blocked with pharmaceuticals to produce a reduced attraction to substances. The authors do a very good job of explaining and anticipating the research progress in anticraving agents for alcohol dependence.

As one of the most experienced physicians identifying and studying physician addicts before and after treatment, Dr. Ray Pomm certainly has pioneered the use of drug testing and has identified testing as an important treatment for addicts. Dr. Pomm understands the importance of using drug testing for diagnosis, prevention, and treatment monitoring. When abstinence is the outcome desired, as it is in physician addictions, positive urine tests are critical and useful outcome measures. While easily explaining pharmacologic and nonpharmacologic treatments, abstinence approaches, and the 12 steps, the authors are equally comfortable with the office treatment of opioid addicts with buprenorphine or naltrexone or methadone. It is so refreshing to see treatments presented impartially in an evidenced base-framework of balancing clinical experience, options, and outcomes. The authors also clearly understand polydrug use and comorbidity. Both are important in the world today where the majority of current cigarette smokers also have a primary psychiatric disease, usually depression or schizophrenia. Being comfortable treating the complete patient is a tall order, but the authors provide helpful advice to make this more likely to happen.

Therefore, it is a great pleasure to write this foreword to Ray and Heidi Pomm's *Management of the Addicted Patient in Primary Care*. I have known Ray Pomm for more than 25 years as a physician expert in addictive disease. Heidi Pomm is a family practitioner mentor and teacher, clinician, and specialist in behavioral treatments for addiction. Together, they have spent their careers thinking about the issues that comprise this text. They have crafted a comprehensive, yet primary care physician-friendly textbook. One challenge to anyone who tries to write a textbook for primary care physicians, the front line and ground zero in the challenge of early detection and prompt nonhospital treatment, is to balance everything that we know about addiction with everything that the practicing physician needs to know to help the patient in the office. Pomm and Pomm's text describes the important core knowledge in addiction medicine and provides a "how to" approach to intervention and treatment that was possible for them to achieve by utilizing vast clinical experience. This book is easy to read and as up to date as any text. Their goal is to improve the education of physicians to the point that they are comfortable and competent treating abusers and addicts. This is a critical mission and attainable if we energize and reemphasize undergraduate and graduate training in addiction medicine as an essential core in compulsory medical education.

Mark S. Gold, MD
Distinguished Professor and Chief
McKnight Brain Institute
Departments of Psychiatry, Neuroscience, Anesthesiology,
Community Health, and Family Medicine
Division of Addiction Medicine

Preface

Whether you like it or not, it is inevitable. You will be (or are) treating alcoholics and addicts who are showing either overt, or covert, symptoms of their disease. In fact, a large number of patients who will seek your help are struggling with substance use disorders; yet the medical establishment is still failing in large numbers to diagnose {addictive disease} in their patients.

Adults and adolescents with substance use disorders (SUD) are likely to be the most difficult patients you will see in your practice. Common physician reactions to these patients include anger, frustration, disgust, and apathy—emotions which may cause the physician to misdiagnose or fail to recognize substance abuse in these patients.

In a survey by The National Center on Addiction and Substance Abuse at Columbia University (CASA), it was demonstrated that 94 percent of primary care physicians failed to include substance abuse among the five diagnoses they offered when presented with early symptoms of alcohol abuse in an adult patient. Furthermore, these researchers found that 41 percent of pediatricians failed to diagnose illegal drug use even when presented with a classic description of a drug-abusing adolescent patient. Some of the greatest barriers to accurate diagnosis appear to be time constraints and patient dishonesty about use. In addition, skepticism about the success of treatment of addicts among physicians appears to be common. Taken together, it appears that it is more necessary than ever for physicians to have the knowledge and skills to appropriately address this population (Califano, 1998; Miller & Sheppard, 1999). In an attempt to fill some of the knowledge-based deficits, it is expected that this book will give you the necessary skills to accurately recognize, diagnose and treat your patients with substance use disorders.

First and foremost, it is important to remember that, when treating patients with addictive illness, ignorance is NOT bliss! In actuality, ignorance only leads to more suffering—for both your patient and yourself. Specifically, this book has been developed to help the primary-care physician deal with patients with substance-use disorders. Because you are reading this book, you probably have a few of these patients in your practice and, by now, you may be experiencing a great deal of frustration because of their behaviors. However, chances are, you never received much (if any) formal training in the area of addiction and you may feel ill-equipped to evaluate and manage these extremely difficult patients. You are not alone! Even the very best physicians can become fed up when it comes to treating alcoholic/addicted patients. By reading this "user-friendly" book, we believe you will gain important and necessary skills which can aid in helping you to feel more in control and less distressed when working with your addicted patient population. It is expected that through the information presented in this book, you will:

- Become more knowledgeable about the latest findings regarding the pathophysiology and genetic factors involved in the development of a substance use disorder (SUD);
- Gain greater skills regarding accurate diagnosis of substance use, abuse and dependence;
- Gain greater expertise in utilizing both pharmacologic and nonpharmacologic interventions that can be administered in an office-based setting to treat your addicted patients.

How to Use This Book

Following this introductory section, Chapter One focuses on the spectrum of addiction; i.e. definitions, a discussion of the "disease model," pathophysiology and genetics, and common drugs of abuse. In Chapter Two, we describe "who" the addicted patient is and the underlying psychological processes common in addictive illness. Twelve-step programs, such as Alcoholics and Narcotics Anonymous, are also discussed in this chapter. Chapter Three provides information about how to assess the presence of SUD, utilizing a variety of instruments, as well as how to obtain a reliable substance abuse history. In Chapter Four, you will find a detailed overview of office-based pharmacologic approaches to managing your patients with SUD. Also in this chapter, we have included definitive parameters to help guide your decision-making regarding your patient's need for inpatient versus outpatient detoxification. Chapter Five introduces brief, effective nonpharmacologic strategies, based on both cognitive-behavioral therapy and motivational interviewing, which you can utilize in an office-based setting. Finally, Chapter Six provides case presentations and algorithms which we feel will aid you in gaining additional insight into these complex patients.

A common slogan in the 12 Step programs is, "First Things First." The development of knowledge and skills within a specific domain first requires a basic & empathic understanding regarding the nature of the problem at hand; hence, we will now move on to discuss the spectrum of addictive disease.

Heidi Allespach Pomm, PhD
Raymond M. Pomm, MD

References

1. The CASA National Survey of Primary Care Physicians and Patients. The National Center on Addiction and Substance Abuse at Columbia University (CASA) 2000.
2. Califano JA Jr. Substance abuse and addiction–the need to know. Am J Public Health. 1998 Jan;88(1):9–11.
3. Miller NS, Sheppard LM. The role of the physician in addiction prevention and treatment. Psychiatr Clin North Am. 1999 Jun;22(2):489–505.

Contents

Contents

1. Spectrum of Addiction

One of the most difficult concepts for many primary care physicians to accept is that addiction is a disease. This thought naturally dispels the idea that people who experience the diagnosed disorder of substance dependence have a choice. Actually, once addiction is manifest in an individual, willpower is no longer a viable hypothesis. At this point, "saying no" does not work (although people diagnosed with substance abuse might still have the ability to choose). Basically, there comes a time when the psychosocial, genetic, biophysiologic and the individual's coping mechanisms have set the stage for a switch to be turned on that starts the disease process, a process that cannot be cured but that can definitely be arrested and brought into remission.

When the disease of addiction manifests in the body, it is no different from any other disease: (1) the illness can be described; (2) the course of the illness is predictable and progressive; (3) the disease is primary; that is, it is not just a symptom of an underlying disorder; (4) it is permanent; and (5) it is terminal. If left untreated, it results in premature death. In fact, the American Psychiatric Association began in 1965 to use the term *disease* to describe alcoholism, and the American Medical Association followed suit in 1966. In 1983, the American Society of Addiction Medicine published a policy statement relating to alcoholism being a primary disease. Essentially, all major specialty organizations that work with the drug/alcohol-addicted population are now in agreement about the disease model of addiction.

We might not know the etiology, but science has not determined the exact etiology of most diseases, including the more common ones, such as hypertension and diabetes mellitus. Yet we do not blame hypertensive or diabetic patients for their diseases in the way that we blame alcoholics/addicts for their illnesses. It seems so much easier to be less judgmental when treating the other types of patients.

Until you accept the disease model of addiction, it is much more difficult to see your patients who are suffering with chemical dependency through objective eyes. As a primary care physician, especially because you are on the front line, you may be more prone to feelings of frustration and anger when confronted with an individual you believe can just "put the substance down." Thoughts such as "why doesn't he or she just stop" or "I can't believe he or she continues using drugs despite all he or she has been through" can interfere with appropriate intervention and treatment planning. Although many professionals are susceptible to the same feelings, the primary care physician often sees this type of patient much earlier in the course of the illness, and a significant relationship may have already been developed (unless a *drug seeker* has just dropped by for your professional services). In addition, beyond the relationship with your patient, you often have a relationship with the family and have also been influenced by their denial system.

If you have not yet accepted the argument favoring the disease model of addiction, the challenge that the authors have is to help convince you that your addicted patients actually do have a primary physical disorder (of course, if you already accept this idea, you may still find this material useful and worth perusing). It is necessary to review some basic neurobiology, epidemiology, genetics, and definitions as a preliminary to the overall discussion of addition.

Neurobiology of Addiction

In order to have a disease, the underlying premise must be that a normally functioning aspect of one's physiology has gone awry. The *normal* part of our physiology that underlies addiction is also found in the manifestation of our need for nurturing, food, fluids, and our desire for sex. Activation in all of these circumstances is mediated through the brain's reward pathway. Basically, addiction hijacks this pathway.

The reward pathway of the brain is called the *mesocorticolimbic area*. The structures in this area include the medial forebrain bundle, the nucleus accumbens (NA), the ventral tegmental area (VTA), and the medial prefrontal cortex (PFC). Dopaminergic, serotonergic, glutamatergic, and gamma-aminobutyric acid (GABA)-ergic neurons are the major neurotransmitters involved. As a basic but central example, neurons in the VTA contain dopamine, which is released in the NA and the PFC. Figure 1.1A–C presents this pathway.

The very fact that the needs for nurturing, food, fluid, and sex are mediated through the same brain region as addiction makes for a complicated scenario. We have all seen examples of similar processes but through different presentations. Food and sexual addictions are problems to which we have all been exposed. These disorders are a little more complicated to treat because we need both food and sex for survival (food for the individual and sex for the species). We propose that humans do not need alcohol, pain killers, or anti-anxiety drugs to survive (although this might be a difficult idea for the addict to accept when he or she is in the depths of illness). The bottom line is, the driving forces for satiety and the experience of satiety are "normal" and are also mediated via the VTA, NA, and PFC. Obviously, something is wrong when we cannot become satiated (food, sex, or drugs/alcohol). In fact, recent research by Bechara (1) has revealed that the body responds to drug withdrawal much like it responds to hunger in that hunger can be conceptualized as a type of withdrawal. Hence, substance withdrawal results in increased motivation to use drugs in the same manner that hunger results in an increased motivation to eat (1).

As we learned in medical school, neurotransmitters are required for neurophysiologic functioning. As previously mentioned, dopamine, serotonin, glutamate, and GABA are the primary neurotransmitters associated with these pathways. Figure 1.2 details the essential elements of the dopaminergic and

Brain Reward:
Nucleus Accumbens (NA)

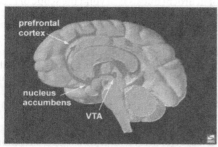

- The "reward center" of the brain.
- Integrates VTA (dopamine) and PFC (glutamine) inputs to determine motivatioinal output.
  – Incentive (appetitive)
  – Reward (consummatory)

A

Brain Reward:
Ventral Temental Area (VTA)

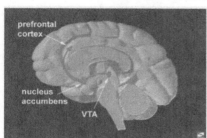

- Location of dopamine cell bodies
- Projects to nucleus accumbens (reward center) and prefrontal cortex (executive control)

B

Brain Reward:
Prefrontal Cortex (PFC)

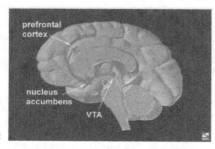

- Exerts executive control over midbrain structures
- "Conscience"
- "Mind"

C

Figure 1.1. (A–C) Brain reward pathways. (From http://www.nida.nih.gov/pubs/teaching/Teaching2/Teaching3.html.)

serotonergic pathways. In addition, medical science has also identified the specific regions of this brain area that are affected by different substances (Figure 1.3).

An in-depth discussion of neurochemicals is beyond the scope of this book. However, for review purposes, let us briefly look at the roles of most of the neurochemical players known to date:

- Dopamine: all drugs of abuse, pleasure (VTA and NA mediated)
- Endogenous opioids (endorphins, etc.): all drugs of abuse; reward, pleasure; possibly involved in the communication between the NA and the PFC
- Norepinephrine: stimulants
- Serotonin: hallucinogens
- GABA: sedatives and alcohol
- Glutamate: N-methyl-D-aspartic acid; withdrawal and stimulation

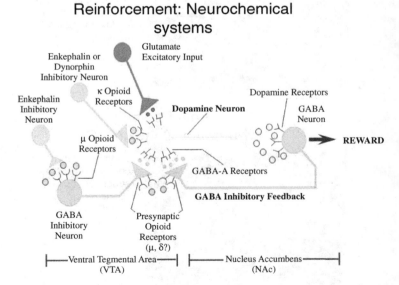

Figure 1.2. Dopamine and serotonin pathways. VTA, ventral tegmental area. (Courtesy of Glen R. Hanson, PhD, DDS, University of Utah, Salt Lake City; casat.unr.edu/docs/ATTC_Las_Vegas.ppt.)

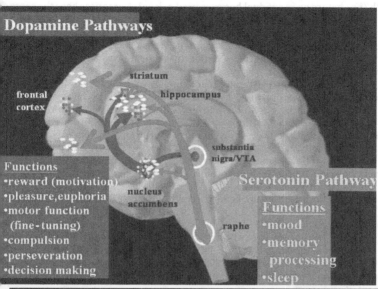

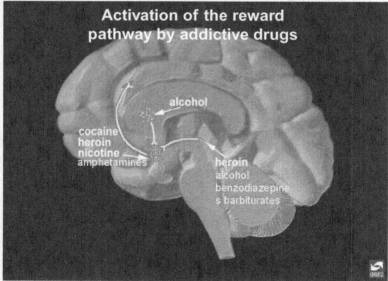

Figure 1.3. Activation of the brain reward pathway by addictive drugs. (From www.drugabuse.gov/pubs/teaching/teaching4/Teaching2.html.)

The brain has receptors for all drugs of abuse, receptors that are present from birth (i.e., before an individual has ever used a drug). Narcotics share the same mu receptors with our bodily produced endogenous opioids. Our bodies even have marijuana receptors, CB1 and CB2 (2). We actually produce an endogenous cannabinoid ligand called *anandamide*. We each appear to have the very best, most efficient, and inexpensive pharmaceutical company—right in our own heads.

Let us also briefly review pharmacokinetics and bioavailability as they relate to addiction (more will be said about these subjects when we discuss specific drugs). Simply stated, *the shorter the half-life and the more rapid the onset of action, the greater is the addictive potential of a drug.* Intuitively, most people assume that the fastest way to move a drug into the body is intravenously. In actuality, rate of absorption, from fastest to slowest route of administration, is as follows: smoking, intravenous, intramuscular, and by mouth. Hence, smoking a drug, such as cocaine, gets one higher faster than shooting the substance into one's veins.

Although both authors are concerned about the rate of substance abuse in the general population, R.M.'s biggest concern right now has to do with the 10%–15% of physicians who have this disease and who may be reading this book. Is their reading the above paragraph going to increase their craving? Just the thought of using drugs can raise the dopamine levels in the NA of an addict or alcoholic (3), and physicians are at least as vulnerable as the general population (4). We now turn to the epidemiologic and genetic underpinnings of the disease of addiction.

Epidemiology of Addiction

A brief summary of recently confirmed epidemiologic facts is presented; the reader can find full information from the following organizations: National Institute of Drug Abuse, National Institute on Alcohol Abuse and Alcoholism, and Substance Abuse and Mental Health Services Administration.

- The lifetime prevalence of having either alcohol abuse or dependence is 13.3%. Lifetime prevalence of alcohol abuse is 12.5% for men and 6.4% for women; lifetime prevalence of alcohol dependence is 20.1% for men and 8.2% for women.
- Benzodiazepines are often used in primary care (5)—10% of adults have exposure to these medications in any given year. From 2% to 4% of overall substance abuse by adults is due mainly to benzodiazepines.
- In 2000, the National Household Survey on Drug Abuse found that 11.2% of the U.S. population over 12 years of age reported ever using cocaine; 1.5% reported using in the past year, and 0.5% reported using within the

past month. Seven percent of drug-abusing individuals reported abuse of other stimulants.

- For DSM-IV-TR (text revision of the *Diagnostic and Statistical Manual of Mental Disorders*, fourth edition), Cannabis Use (*not* Disorder), life-time prevalence was 50% in the 26–34-year-old age group and 32% in all ages. Highest cannabis use in the past year was 24% in the 18–25-year-old age group and 9% in all ages. Past month data revealed 5% use in all ages and 13% in the 18–25-year-old group.
- Some subgroups within racial/ethnic minorities may be at greater risk of substance abuse, and there is little question that these risks are related to observed health disparities among these populations.
- There are approximately 1,000,000 opioid addicts in the United States, and the majority are between 20 and 39 years of age; however, there has been an increase in use among 15–21 year olds. In fact, hydrocodone preparations have recently been found to be second only to marijuana as drugs abused amongst highschool students.
- In 2000, 23% of individuals smoked cigarettes (19% daily and 4% occasionally). The percentage of ex-smokers in this study was 22%; 55% of respondents reported that they had never smoked.

Prescription drug abuse is a growing problem. Hydrocodone, oxycodone, and methadone (not from methadone maintenance clinics) are a large concern for the boards of medicine and the state legislatures around the country. Even fentanyl abuse is becoming a significant problem. Throw in the commonly found abuse of prescription Xanax, and one has a very deadly combination. The question can be raised: Why are some individuals more likely to develop the disease of addiction than others?

Genetics of Addiction

An abundance of literature supports a strong genetic influence in alcoholism (as of yet, not as many studies have been performed related to drug addiction, but alcohol is one of the oldest known drugs). The most compelling evidence to date appears to be found in studies focusing on twins. In one study, the individuals included were raised apart from at least one alcoholic parent or alcoholic surrogate parent. Those born to the alcoholic parent were significantly more likely to develop alcoholism compared with those born to the surrogate (6).

Researchers in Sweden identified a far greater rate of alcoholism among male monozygotic twins versus male dizygotic twins: 60% versus 39% (7). These numbers have been closely replicated in several studies up to 1995 (8). Table 1.1 provides further study results for specific drugs with an additional comparison of male versus female subjects.

Table 1.1. Addiction is a heritable disorder: twin studies.

Drug	Male subjects	Female subjects
Heroin (opiates)	54% (Tsuang et al., 1996)[15]	
Sedatives	87% (Kendler et al., 2000)[16]	
Marijuana	33% (Tsuang et al., 1996)[15]	79% (Kendler and Prescott, 1998)[18]
	58% (Kendler et al., 2000)[16]	
Cocaine	44% (Tsuang et al., 1996)[15]	81% (Kendler et al., 1999)[19]
	79% (Kendler et al., 2000)[16]	
Hallucinogens	79% (Kendler et al., 2000)[16]	
Nicotine	53% (Carmelli et al., 1990)[17]	72% (Kendler et al., 1999)[19]

Source: Pollock JD. Genetics and Addiction (Power Point Presentation). Division of Neuroscience & Behavioral Research, National Institute on Drug Abuse, National Institutes of Health, Department of Health and Human Services (http://www.nida.nih.gov/about/organization/nacda/powerpoint/JPGenetics03council).

Multiple studies have shown that the rate of alcoholism is significantly greater among children of alcoholic parents than among children of nonalcoholic parents. Children born to alcoholic parents have a three to four times greater risk of developing alcoholism (9).

Higuchi et al. (10) published an interesting study relating to alcohol metabolism that is similar to an Antabuse reaction (Figure 1.4). Antabuse acts by reducing the activity of aldehyde dehydrogenase (ALDH), which causes a buildup of acetaldehyde resulting in the Antabuse reaction. Some of the classic symptoms include flushing, gastrointestinal distress, and cardiac effects (see Chapter 4 for a more in-depth discussion). In the study by Higuchi et al. (10), it was found that Japanese men with the ALDH2 genotype have a decreased incidence of alcoholism. In other words, they have a "built-in" Antabuse-like reaction.

Women tend to experience a greater toxic effect from alcohol. They have less alcohol dehydrogenase in their stomach lining (where a significant amount of alcohol begins its metabolism). Therefore, a greater amount of alcohol enters their bloodstream compared to men (11). In fact, a nice review article regarding women and alcohol was published by the National Institute on Alcohol Abuse and Alcoholism (12).

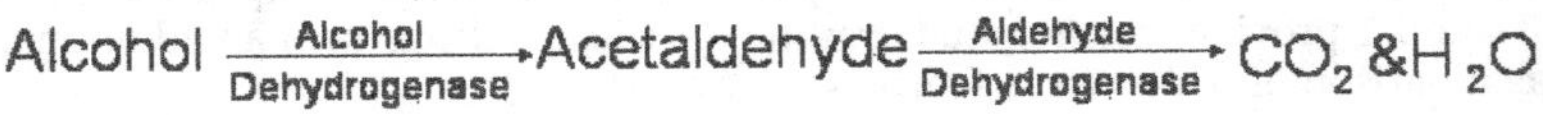

$$\text{Alcohol} \xrightarrow[\text{Dehydrogenase}]{\text{Alcohol}} \text{Acetaldehyde} \xrightarrow[\text{Dehydrogenase}]{\text{Aldehyde}} CO_2 \,\&\, H_2O$$

Figure 1.4. Metabolic pathway of alcohol.

There is so much more evidence relating to genetic implications. According to recent genomic studies, two chromosomes, 17 and 2, have been implicated in heavy opioid use and alcohol dependence, respectively (13). There also appears to be genetic influences in choice of drugs, addiction, and withdrawal seizures. In addition, there may be genetic involvement in the development of Wernicke-Korsakoff syndrome, cirrhosis, and pancreatitis. However, these issues are beyond the scope of this book, and we refer readers to a textbook on addiction medicine for a more comprehensive review (14).

At this point, we hope some headway has been made convincing those readers who had not accepted the disease concept that there is, in fact, a disease process underlying patients' addictions.

Definitions

We all use the terms *addict* and *abuser*. In fact, in our review of research articles, both throughout our careers and in preparation for the writing of this book, little differentiation is made between these two terms. However, the terms are specific, and we define them for consistency within the context of this book.

The term *addict* is used for someone who suffers with an addiction and also someone who is substance (chemically) dependent. The American Society of Addiction Medicine (ASAM) defines addiction as a "disease process characterized by the continued use of a specific psychoactive substance despite physical, psychological or social harm." ASAM uses the term "dependence" in three different ways: "(1) physical dependence, a physiological state of adaptation to a specific psychoactive substance characterized by the emergence of a withdrawal syndrome during abstinence, which may be relieved in total or in part by readministration of the substance; (2) psychological dependence, a subjective sense of need for a specific psychoactive substance, either for its positive effects or to avoid negative effects associated with its abstinence; and (3) one category of psychoactive substance use disorder" (14).

The book used most consistently to determine the presence of a substance use disorder is the DSM-IV-TR. For diagnostic purposes, it gives specific criteria for the diagnosis of substance dependence (the following diagnostic criteria are reprinted with permission from the *Diagnostic and Statistical Manual of Mental Disorders*, Copyright © 2000, American Psychiatric Association):

A maladaptive pattern of substance use, leading to clinically significant impairment or distress, as manifest by three (or more) of the following, occurring at any time in the same 12-month period:

(1) tolerance, as defined by either of the following:
   (a) a need for markedly increased amounts of the substance to achieve intoxication or the desired effect
   (b) markedly diminished effect with continued use of the same amount of the substance
(2) withdrawal, as manifested by either of the following:
   (a) the characteristic withdrawal syndrome for the substance (refer to Criteria A and B of the criteria sets for Withdrawal from the specific Substances)
   (b) the same (or a closely related) substance is taken to relieve or avoid withdrawal symptoms
(3) the substance is often taken in larger amounts or over a longer period than was intended
(4) there is a persistent desire or unsuccessful efforts to cut down or control substance use
(5) a great deal of time is spent in activities necessary to obtain the substance (e.g., visiting multiple doctors or driving long distances), use the substance (e.g., chain-smoking), or recover from its effects
(6) important social, occupational, or recreational activities are given up or reduced because of substance use
(7) the substance use is continued despite knowledge of having a persistent or recurrent physical or psychological problem that is likely to have been caused or exacerbated by the substance (e.g., current cocaine use despite recognition of cocaine-induced depression, or continued drinking despite recognition that an ulcer was made worse by alcohol consumption).

For further clarification, we fine-tune the previously mentioned definitions through an example: If, through the course of pain management, your patient becomes dependent on the prescribed narcotic, the patient has developed a dependence that will need to be handled via a specific detoxification schedule (if and when appropriate). The patient is not necessarily an addict. An addict would have to display the required number of the DSM-IV-TR diagnostic criteria in order to be labeled substance dependent (an addict).

Another term that should be defined is *pseudoaddiction*. Patients with a pseudoaddiction can be particularly difficult. They are often dramatic and demanding. In fact, these patients can act just like an addict who is on the verge of being out of control (or might actually be out of control). This scenario often occurs when the individual is undertreated, that is, the dosing schedule of a particular medication or the potency of the drug chosen is not adequate. In either case, if the patient is not an addict, then when the medication or medical problem is corrected, the behavior abates.

To further illustrate the differences between the terms *addict* and *pseudo-addict*, imagine that you have two patients—both of whom are physically dependent on opioids and who both complain of chronic low back pain. Both of these patients went through a medical detoxification and thus were no longer opioid dependent. Now let us imagine that we were magically able to take away the pain in their lower backs. The pseudoaddict would no longer have any interest in taking narcotic medications; to him, the pain was the primary issue, and, now that his pain is gone, he no longer needs (or wants) the narcotics. The addict, on the other hand, would still want the opioid medication, because, for him, the drug—not the pain—is the primary issue.

The term *substance abuse*, according to DSM-IV-TR, is defined by the diagnostic criteria that should be used to help in the differential diagnosis (diagnostic criteria are reprinted with permission from the *Diagnostic and Statistical Manual of Mental Disorders*, Copyright © 2000, American Psychiatric Association):

A. A maladaptive pattern of substance use leading to clinically significant impairment or distress, as manifest by one (or more) of the following, occurring within a 12-month period:
   (1) recurrent substance use resulting in a failure to fulfill major role obligations at work, school, or home (e.g., repeated absences or poor work performance related to substance use, substance-related absences, suspensions or expulsions from school; neglect of children or household)
   (2) recurrent substance use in situations in which it is physically hazardous (e.g., driving an automobile or operating a machine when impaired by substance use)
   (3) recurrent substance-related legal problems (e.g., arrests for substance-related disorderly conduct)
   (4) continued substance use despite having persistent or recurrent social or interpersonal problems caused or exacerbated by the effects of the substance (e.g., arguments with spouse about consequences of intoxication, physical fights)
B. The symptoms have never met the criteria for Substance Dependence for this class of substance.

Please note that criterion B is important.

We, the authors, tend to cheat a little when it comes to remembering the previously mentioned criteria for substance abuse in that we do not go through the entire list. We remember that there are at least two significant substance-related consequences for an individual within a 12-month period of time in order to receive a diagnosis of substance abuse.

The differences between abuse and dependence are important. Those with abuse (who do not go on to exhibit symptoms of addictive illness) tend to have normal brain chemistry. They are likely to stop as consequences progress; it is usually self-limited. As stated in the first paragraph of this chapter, those who have substance abuse can still "say no"; they are in control of their drug use. Those with dependence are controlled by their drug use secondary to an abnormally functioning mesocorticolimbic area of their brain.

To conclude this chapter, Table 1.2 lists commonly abused drugs, their commercial and street names, their U.S. Drug Enforcement Administration schedule classification, how they are administered, and their intoxication effects and potential health consequences.

Table 1.2. Commonly abused drugs.

Substance: category and name	Examples of *commercial* and street names	Schedule*/how administered[†]	*Intoxication effects/potential health consequences*
Cannabinoids			*Euphoria, slowed thinking and reaction time, confusion, impaired balance and coordination/cough, frequent respiratory infections; impaired memory and learning; increased heart rate, anxiety; panic attacks; tolerance, addiction*
Hashish	Boom, chronic, gangster, hash, hash oil, hemp	I/swallowed, smoked	
Marijuana	Blunt, dope, ganja, grass, herb, joints, Mary Jane, pot, reefer, sinsemilla, skunk, weed	I/swallowed, smoked	
Depressants			*Reduced anxiety; feeling of well-being; lowered inhibitions; slowed pulse and breathing; lowered blood pressure; poor concentration/fatigue; confusion; impaired coordination, memory, judgment; addiction; respiratory depression and arrest, death*
Barbiturates	*Amytal, Nembutal, Seconal, phenobarbital;* barbs, reds, red birds, phennies, tooies, yellows, yellow jackets	II, III, V/injected, swallowed	*Also for barbiturates—sedation, drowsiness/depression, unusual excitement, fever, irritability, poor judgment, slurred speech, dizziness, life-threatening withdrawal*
Benzodiazepines (other than flunitrazepam)	*Ativan, Halcion, Librium, Valium, Xanax;* candy, downers, sleeping pills, tranks	IV/swallowed, injected	*Also for benzodiazepines— sedation, drowsiness/dizziness*

(Continued)

Drug	Street names	Schedule/route	Effects
Flunitrazepam‡	Rohypnol; forget-me pill, Mexican Valium, R2, Roche, roofies, roofinol, rope, rophies	IV/swallowed, snorted	Also for flunitrazepam—visual and gastrointestinal disturbances, urinary retention, memory loss for the time under the drug's effects
GHB‡	Gamma-hydroxybutyrate; G, Georgia home boy, grievous bodily harm, liquid ecstasy	I/swallowed	Also for GHB—drowsiness, nausea/vomiting, headache, loss of consciousness, loss of reflexes, seizures, coma, death
Methaqualone	Quaalude, Sopor, Parest; ludes, mandrex, quad, quay	I/injected, swallowed	Also for methaqualone— euphoria/depression, poor reflexes, slurred speech, coma
Dissociative anesthetics			Increased heart rate and blood pressure, impaired motor function/memory loss; numbness; nausea/vomiting
Ketamine	Ketalar SV; cat Valiums, K, Special K, vitamin K	III/injected, snorted, smoked	Also for ketamine—at high doses, delirium, depression, respiratory depression and arrest
PCP and analogs	Phencyclidine; angel dust, boat, hog, love boat, peace pill	I, II/injected, swallowed, smoked	Also for PCP and analogs— possible decrease in blood pressure and heart rate, panic, aggression, violence/loss of appetite, depression
Hallucinogens			Altered states of perception and feeling; nausea; persisting perception disorder (flashbacks)
LSD	Lysergic acid diethylamide; acid, blotter, boomers, cubes, microdot, yellow sunshines	I/swallowed, absorbed through mouth tissues	Also for LSD and mescaline— increased body temperature, heart rate, blood pressure; loss of appetite, sleeplessness, numbness, weakness, tremors. for LSD—persistent mental disorders
Mescaline	Buttons, cactus, mesc, peyote	I/swallowed, smoked	
Psilocybin	Magic mushroom, purple passion, shrooms	I/swallowed	Also for psilocybin— nervousness, paranoia

Table 1.2. *Continued*

Substance: category and name	Examples of *commercial and* street names	Schedule*/how administered[†]	*Intoxication effects/potential health consequences*
Opioids and morphine derivatives			*Pain relief, euphoria, drowsiness/nausea, constipation, confusion, sedation, respiratory depression and arrest, tolerance, addiction, unconsciousness, coma, death*
Codeine	*Empirin with Codeine, Fiorinal with Codeine, Robitussin A–C, Tylenol with Codeine;* Captain Cody, Cody, schoolboy; (with glutethimide) doors & fours, loads, pancakes and syrup	II, III, IV/injected, swallowed	*Also for codeine—less analgesia, sedation, and respiratory depression than morphine*
Fentanyl and fentanyl analogs	*Actiq, Duragesic, Sublimaze;* Apache, China girl, China white, dance fever, friend, goodfella, jackpot, murder 8, TNT, Tango and Cash	I, II/injected, smoked, snorted	
Heroin	*Diacetylmorphine;* brown sugar, dope, H, horse, junk, skag, skunk, smack, white horse	I/injected, smoked, snorted	*Also for heroin—staggering gait*
Morphine	*Roxanol, Duramorph;* M, Miss Emma, monkey, white stuff	II, III/injected, swallowed, smoked	
Opium	*Laudanum, paregoric;* big O, black stuff, block, gum, hop	II, III, V/swallowed, smoked	
Oxycodone hydrochloride	*OxyContin;* Oxy, OC, killer	II/swallowed, snorted, injected	
Hydrocodone bitartrate, acetaminophen	*Vicodin;* vike, Watson-387	II/swallowed	

			Increased heart rate, blood pressure, metabolism; feelings of exhilaration, energy, increased mental alertness/rapid or irregular heart beat; reduced appetite, weight loss, heart failure, nervousness, insomnia
Stimulants			
Amphetamine	*Biphetamine, Dexedrine;* bennies, black beauties, crosses, hearts, LA turnaround, speed, truck drivers, uppers	II/injected, swallowed, smoked, snorted	*Also for amphetamine*—rapid breathing/tremor, loss of coordination; irritability, anxiousness, restlessness, delirium, panic, paranoia, impulsive behavior, aggressiveness, tolerance, addiction, psychosis
Cocaine	*Cocaine hydrochloride;* blow, bump, C, candy, Charlie, coke, crack, flake, rock, snow, toot	II/injected, smoked, snorted	*Also for cocaine*—increased temperature/chest pain, respiratory failure, nausea, abdominal pain, strokes, seizures, headaches, malnutrition, panic attacks
MDMA	Adam, clarity, ecstasy, Eve, lover's speed, peace, STP, X, XTC	I/swallowed	*Also for MDMA*—mild hallucinogenic effects, increased tactile sensitivity, empathic feelings/impaired memory and learning, hyperthermia, cardiac toxicity, renal failure, liver toxicity
Methamphetamine	*Desoxyn;* chalk, crank, crystal, fire, glass, go fast, ice, meth, speed	II/injected, swallowed, smoked, snorted	*Also for methamphetamine*— aggression, violence, psychotic behavior/memory loss, cardiac and neurologic damage; impaired memory and learning, tolerance, addiction
Methylphenidate (safe and effective for treatment of ADHD)	*Ritalin;* JIF, MPH, R-ball, Skippy, the smart drug, vitamin R	II/injected, swallowed, snorted	
Nicotine	Cigarettes, cigars, smokeless tobacco, snuff, spit tobacco, bidis, chew	Not scheduled/smoked, snorted, taken in snuff and spit tobacco	*Also for nicotine*—additional effects attributable to tobacco exposure, adverse pregnancy outcomes, chronic lung disease, cardiovascular disease, stroke, cancer, tolerance, addiction

(Continued)

Table 1.2. *Continued*

Substance: category and name	Examples of *commercial and street names*	Schedule*/how administered[†]	*Intoxication effects/potential health consequences*
Other compounds			
Anabolic steroids	*Anadrol, Oxandrin, Durabolin, Depo-Testosterone, Equipoise;* roids, juice	III/injected, swallowed, applied to skin	*No intoxication effects*/hypertension, blood clotting and cholesterol changes, liver cysts and cancer, kidney cancer, hostility and aggression, acne; in adolescents, premature stoppage of growth; in males, prostate cancer, reduced sperm production, shrunken testicles, breast enlargement; in females, menstrual irregularities, development of beard and other masculine characteristics
Inhalants	*Solvents (paint thinners, gasoline, glues), gases (butane, propane, aerosol propellants, nitrous oxide), nitrites (isoamyl, isobutyl, cyclohexyl);* laughing gas, poppers, snappers, whippets	Not scheduled/inhaled through nose or mouth	*Stimulation, loss of inhibition; headache; nausea or vomiting; slurred speech, loss of motor coordination; wheezing*/unconsciousness, cramps, weight loss, muscle weakness, depression, memory impairment, damage to cardiovascular and nervous systems, sudden death

Note: ADHD, attention deficit hyperactivity disorder; MDMA, 3,4-methylenedioxymethamphetamine.

*U.S. Drug Enforcement Administration Schedule I and II drugs have a high potential for abuse. They require greater storage security and have a quota on manufacturing, among other restrictions. Schedule I drugs are available for research only and have no approved medical use; Schedule II drugs are available only by prescription (nonrefillable) and require a form for ordering. Schedule III and IV drugs are available by prescription, may have five refills in 6 months, and may be ordered orally. Most Schedule V drugs are available over the counter.

[†] Taking drugs by injection can increase the risk of infection through needle contamination with staphylococci, human immunodeficiency virus, hepatitis, and other organisms.

[‡] Associated with sexual assaults.

Source: From http://www.nida.nih.gov/DrugPages/DrugsofAbuse.html.

References

1. Bechara A. Decision making, impulse control and loss of willpower to resist drugs: a neurocognitive perspective. Nat Neurosci 2005;8(11):1458–1463.

2. Howlett AC. Pharmacology of cannabinoid receptors. Annu Rev Pharmacol Toxicol 1995;35:607–634.

3. Le Foll B, Frances H, Diaz J, Schwartz JC, Sokoloff P. Role of the dopamine D3 receptor in reactivity to cocaine-associated cues in mice. Eur J Neurosci 2002;15(12):2016–2026.

4. Brandt JF, Brandt JM, Pomm RM, Frost-Pineda K, Gold MS. Florida Impaired Physicians: Longitudinal, Urine Testing Confirmed, 5-Year Outcomes Study. First Prize Physician Research Award, Florida Academy of Family Physicians, Destin, FL, November 7–8 2001.

5. Piper A Jr. Addiction to benzodiazepines—how common? Arch Fam Med 1995;4(11): 964–970.

6. Schuckit MA, Goodwin DW, Winokur GA. A study of alcoholism in half-siblings. Am J Psychiatry 1972;128:1132–1136.

7. Kaij L. Studies on the Etiology and Sequelae of Abuse of Alcohol. Lund, Sweden: University of Lund Press; 1960.

8. Prescott CA, Kendler KS. Twin study design. Alcohol Health Res World 1995;19:200–205.

9. Schuckit MA. Biological vulnerability to alcoholism. J Consult Clin Psychol 1987;55:1–9.

10. Higuchi S, Matsushita S, Murayama M, Takagi S, Hayashida M. Alcohol and aldehyde dehydrogenase polymorphisms and the risk for alcoholism. Am J Psychiatry 1995; 152(8):1219–1221.

11. Frezza M, di Padova C, Pozzato G, Terpin M, Baraona E, Lieber CS. High blood alcohol levels in women: the role of decreased gastric alcohol dehydrogenase activity and first-pass metabolism. N Engl J Med 1990;322(2):95–99.

12. Alcohol Alert. National Institute on Alcohol Abuse and Alcoholism. No. 10 PH 290, October 1990.

13. Gelernter J, et al. Genomewide linkage scan for opioid dependence and related traits. Am J Hum Genet 2005;78:759–769.

14. Graham AW, Schultz TK. Principles of Addiction Medicine, 2nd ed. Chevy Chase, MD: American Society of Addiction Medicine; 1998.

15. Tsuang MT, Lyons MJ, Eisen SA, Goldberg J, True W, Lin N, Meyer JM, Toomey R, Faraone SV, Eaves L. Genetic influences on DSM-III-R drug abuse and dependence: a study of 3,372 twin pairs. Am J Med Genet 1996;67:473–477.

16. Kendler KS, Karkowski LM, Neale MC, Prescott CA. Illicit psychoactive substance use, heavy use, abuse, and dependence in a US population-based sample of male twins. Arch Gen Psychiatry 2000;57:261–269.

17. Carmelli D, Swan GE, Robinette D, Fabsitz RR. Heritability of substance use in the NAS-NRC Twin Registry. Acta Genet Med Gemellol (Roma) 1990;39:91–98.

18. Kendler KS, Prescott CA. Cannabis use, abuse, and dependence in a population-based sample of female twins. Am J Psychiatry 1998;155:1016–1022.

19. Kendler KS, Karkowski L, Prescott CA. Hallucinogen, opiate, sedative and stimulant use and abuse in a population-based sample of female twins. Acta Psychiatr Scand 1999;99:368–376.

2. The Addicted Patient

Who *is* the addicted patient? We all know how addicted patients behave, but *why* do they behave in this manner? In Chapter 1, we describe the physiology of addiction, and in Chapter 3 we present ways to identify addicted patients. However, also understanding who addicted patients really are and why they act in seemingly "insane" ways is of the utmost importance when managing this type of patient in the office-based setting. Three aspects of the addicted patient are especially noteworthy: 1) addiction as a fear-based illness, 2) psychosocial functioning, and 3) the process of denial. We discuss these aspects in this chapter as well. What the primary care physician needs to know about 12-step programs, such as Alcoholics Anonymous, Narcotics Anonymous, and Al-Anon.

Addiction Is a Fear-Based Illness

My whole life and thinking was centered around getting drugs in one form or another. I "lived to use and used to live" as they say in AA. I came from a good family and was raised right by parents with really good morals. Yet, by my early '40's, here I was, spending all of my time going from one doctor to another to get narcotics. . . . I couldn't imagine living without them. I mean, how would I cope? So when one doctor told me "No" . . . I got really angry. I guess I felt that he was trying to take away the most important thing in my life . . . the ONLY thing I really could care about in my life. I thought, "How could he do this to me? He is obviously going out of his way to hurt me. How can I ever live without my drugs?"

—John M.

In order to help your addicted patients, it is necessary to understand that addiction is often referred to as a *fear-based illness*. The addicted patient has an illness in which fear, in the earlier stages, may not be so noticeable—the addict may appear to be self-confident and even a bit grandiose and demanding. However, as the disease of addiction progresses, the underlying fear becomes more and more evident. It may manifest as anger (especially if your patient views you as an obstacle to getting his or her drugs), overt anxiety, manipulation, desperation, depression, and/or hopelessness. Many of our patients have described the historical nature of their fear: "I have always felt different somehow—I never felt as good as others," "I think we addicts are 'high-wired,' anxious people . . . we use drugs to numb us because we feel everything and that really hurts." Your addicted patient is not a bad, weak, or amoralistic person. Addicted patients do not have poor "willpower." The simple fact is that your addicted patients have a disease that, if not arrested, will result in "jails, institutions or death." (1). The essence of this illness is fear. As the addicted patient slips further and further into his or her addiction, after many failed attempts to control or stop his or her alcohol or other drug use, all control is lost, and an overwhelming sense of fear and despair takes over. In the Alcoholics Anonymous (AA) Big Book, the "bible" of AA, this phenomenon is nicely illustrated:

> We alcoholics are men and women who have lost the ability to control our drinking. We know that no real alcoholic *ever* recovers control. All of us felt at times that we were regaining control, but such intervals—usually brief—were inevitably followed by still less control, which led in time to pitiful and incomprehensible demoralization. We are convinced to a man that alcoholics of our type are in the grips of a progressive illness. Over any considerable period, we get worse, never better. (p. 30 [1])

As a primary care physician, you have probably felt frustrated, angry, disappointed—even apathetic—about these types of patients. It may be helpful to know that these patients, especially in the later stages, are usually feeling ashamed, scared, and very angry and disappointed in themselves too. Unfortunately, they will rarely exhibit these emotions; rather, you will likely experience these patients reacting to you in angry, demanding, and/or manipulative ways. We teach our residents to try to detach from the patient's anger or other negative feeling states or behaviors in order to see the fear and desperation that dwell beneath. If you are able to look at the suffering person underneath all of the "lashing out," you may feel less stressed by such difficult patients.

Not personalizing your patient's behaviors can also be useful. Specifically, if you have attempted to help your patient but the patient continues to use substances, despite all you have done, it is important to realize that this has nothing to do with you or with your skill as a physician. The patient is not doing anything to *you*; that is, he or she acts this way with everyone. Addicted patients are on a path and, depending on what stage of change they are in (stages of change are discussed in Chapter 5), will likely continue on that path until the pain and fear finally become severe enough to motivate them to seek recovery. However, while you are not responsible for "making" your patients stop their substance use, there are some strategies you can use to assist them in traversing through these stages a little more quickly. These strategies, along with the definition of each stage of change, are presented in depth in Chapter 5.

The CALMER Approach is another framework that may assist you in managing the distressful feelings that can result from working with difficult patients (2). To summarize, the CALMER Approach offers "six steps to serenity" when treating patients who are problematic. These steps are as follows (2):

Step One: Catalyst (you are only a catalyst for patient change; you are not responsible for *making* the patient change his or her behaviors);

Step Two: Alter (alter your thoughts about your addicted patients in order to alter your feelings about them);

Step Three: Listen, then make a diagnosis (only by engaging in Steps 1 and 2 can you truly "listen" to what your patient is telling you—both verbally and, even more importantly many times, nonverbally. Further, only by listening can you obtain enough accurate information to make the correct diagnosis);

Step Four: Make an agreement with the patient (set appropriate expectations and boundaries with the patient in order to create a plan of action. This may include a contract for narcotic or benzodiazepine use or may involve an agreement from the patient that he or she will attend an AA meeting before the next visit, etc.);

Step Five: Education (educate your addicted patients about the disease and what resources, such as local treatment centers and the 12 Step programs, are available to help them);

Step Six: Reach out (and discuss your feelings with trusted colleagues and friends—it is normal to have "negative" feelings toward addicted patients, and it is important to "vent" them in a healthy manner). (Reprinted with permission from ref. 2.)

Sadly, there are many, many addicted patients who never do find recovery, and many of them die of this illness . . . and the majority of them die alone.

Psychosocial Functioning

When I first started drinking heavily, it was cool and very accepted because everybody partied at college—that was the thing to do, right? When I got into med school, I would only drink on the weekends to let off steam. All of the people I hung out with drank too. But, in my second year, the weekend started moving into Friday and Monday too. My grades started to slip a bit but, most importantly, my relationships with my family and with my old nondrinking friends were getting really strained. My parents obviously knew that something was going on, but I guess they didn't want to confront me. I withdrew from my family and old friends and even stopped going out on the weekends. . . . I just began drinking in my apartment. By my third and fourth years of med school, I was basically a recluse and drank pretty much all the time—except when I was in class. I have no clue how I graduated, but I did . . . no one at school ever knew because I would always make up excuses, "Oh, I have the flu" or "I have been out of town a lot. . . ." It was amazing how they would all believe whatever I told them.

—Paul R., MD

A critical concept to understand when treating a patient with a substance use disorder is that every area of his or her life has been affected by this disease—cognitions, emotions, relationships, health, sexuality, spirituality, and school/work. In Chapter 5, we present a detailed discussion of how to use cognitive-behavioral therapy (CBT) in the office-based setting. However, certain key points about CBT should also be noted here. Cognitive-behavioral therapy theory posits, "We feel what we think." That is, thoughts create feelings, and feelings, in turn, affect physical sensations and behaviors. The patient in active addiction has negative, distorted cognitions that then lead to distressful feelings. These feelings then (in part) lead to the physical sensation of craving, and the patient will engage in behaviors aimed at reduction of this distress, namely, using substances. Negative, distorted cognitions *must* be addressed and replaced, or restructured, with more positive, balanced thoughts if long-term abstinence is to be achieved.

One of the greatest areas of pain for patients in the grips of addiction is the havoc their illness has wreaked upon their close relationships with the people they love. The majority of addicted patients become increasingly isolated and withdrawn as their disease progresses. In addition, family and friends, who may have tried for years to reason, cajole, confront, intervene, coax, and threaten the patient in an effort to get him or her to stop using, usually reach a breaking point where they have to disengage or lose themselves in the chaos and confusion surrounding their addicted loved one. This is why addiction is often referred to as a "family illness." Indeed, addicts' behaviors typically affect those closest to them (family, good friends) first, while school and work are usually the last areas to be affected. The Big Book of AA (which is discussed later in this section) states, "A doctor said to us, 'Years of living with an alcoholic is almost sure to make any (spouse) or child neurotic. The entire family is, to some extent, ill'" (1).

As a primary care physician, one of the most important, and often the most difficult, challenges you may confront will be to treat the patient and his or her family in order to help restore functioning for all the individuals afflicted directly and indirectly by this disease. One way to do this, if the physician is comfortable, is to have a "family conference" with the addicted patient and his or her loved ones. Talking about the "elephant in the room" (i.e., often the patient knows that there is a problem, the family knows that there is a problem, but no one is really talking about the "elephant"—they skirt around it, trying to pretend it does not exist) can be healthy and cathartic and can "plant the seeds" for a future commitment to recovery. Even if the patient is resistant to getting help, communication has been facilitated, and the patient and family now know they have "permission" to discuss this topic with you. If the patient is open to getting further help, then a plan can be discussed and the entire family can be helped to understand what their role is in the recovery process. Of course, referral to a family therapist is also recommended and can be quite beneficial for families in distress. It should be emphasized that the physician must feel comfortable and confident in his or her skills to have an effective conference with the addicted patient and the patient's family members present. These types of visits can become quite combustible, as the family often has a great deal of anger toward the patient. If you do choose to have a family meeting as a first-line intervention, again, referral to a psychologist or family counselor for ongoing psychotherapy is highly recommended. Some general guidelines for how to lead an effective family conference are presented in Chapter 5.

By first addressing the area that usually means the most to the addicted patient—relationships—the other afflicted areas (work, health, etc.) can also begin to be pieced back together, one at a time. Addiction affects every aspect of the addicted person's life and the lives of those around him or her, and all aspects must be addressed in a systematic fashion to assist in long-term recovery. Before any area can be addressed, however, the patient must confront his or her denial and stop using substances.

Denial (Not the River in Egypt)

For so many years, I was able to deny that I had a problem with Xanax. I was able to tell myself, "It's okay . . . my doctor prescribed it," and "Well, I am feeling really anxious right now so I should take twice the dose." Sometimes, lots of times, actually, I took much more than even twice the dose but I was always able to rationalize and justify it. Everyone around me kept telling me that they were worried because I seemed so "out of it" and I would just get really mad at them. What did they know? I was okay—I was in control. Now I realize how truly sick I was. . . . I was totally in denial about my problem with this medication. I wish I had listened to them sooner . . . before I lost my family and most of my friends because of my addiction.

—Jennifer T.

The concept of denial originated with Sigmund Freud's work on the unconscious processes of the mind. Denial is a defense mechanism that manifests as the refusal to acknowledge the existence of unacceptable and/or painful external realities and/or internal thoughts and feelings. In regard to addiction, denial appears to be at its peak during the precontemplative stage (see Chapter 5). The addicted patient denies that he or she has a problem with substances, even though others can clearly see the addict's struggle. When confronted, the addict usually reacts with anger and defensiveness. There is an old saying, "Underneath anger is always fear." Again, it is important to recognize that the addict is terrified, albeit unconsciously, of living life without drugs because that seems, paradoxically, like death. The majority of addicts feel that, without their drug of choice, they will "fall apart" and not be able to cope with anything (on average, most have used drugs or alcohol to cope for most of their lives and do not have the requisite "sober" experience to manage stress without significant help). This terror, then, is expressed as rage when the addict is confronted, and he or she will use any means to continue using because "using" means "living" in the distorted cognitions of the active addict.

Strategies that have been suggested for addicts in the precontemplative and contemplative stages of change are especially useful in addressing denial. One strategy, often used by physicians in primary care but not recommended by these authors, is direct confrontation, or "ordering" the patient to stop using substances. This strategy tends to reinforce denial and resistance—which is obviously the opposite of our intended goal of complete abstinence from all substances. A gentler approach leads to a gradual diminishing of denial and movement toward the next stage of change. These strategies, suggested for patients in the first two stages of change, are detailed in Chapter 5.

What the Primary Care Physician Needs to Know About Alcoholics Anonymous, Narcotics Anonymous, and Al-Anon

> Alcoholics Anonymous is a worldwide fellowship of more than one million men and women who are banded together to solve their common problems and to help fellow sufferers in recovery from that age-old, baffling malady, alcoholism. (p. 3 [3])

The 12 Step programs of AA and Narcotics Anonymous (NA) are undisputedly the best "treatment" options for long-term sobriety/abstinence for your addicted patients and the only modality that offers support for your patients for many years to come (4). Instead of you, as the patient's doctor, being the primary resource in times of crisis, your addicted patients learn to turn first to the 12 Step programs for help. Although the 12 Step programs are not considered formal alcohol and/or drug treatment, their availability and philosophy are aimed at promoting long-term abstinence from all substances. We strongly suggest keeping the phone numbers to AA and NA readily accessible in your office so that you may give them to patients who are ready to make a step toward sobriety. Most local groups of both AA and NA have meeting lists available online that can be printed out and handed to your more motivated patients. When residents rotate with me (H.P.), I require that they attend one AA or NA meeting, as well as an Al-Anon meeting, so that they can then tell their patients what to expect when attending a meeting for the first time.

The addict in distress, whose fear and resistance are at a crescendo, may be very resistant to going to a 12 Step meeting—even though he or she truly wants to stop drinking or using drugs. Common reasons an active addict gives for *not* attending a meeting are: "I don't want to go to AA—everyone is drunk there"; "I have heard that they make you stand up at a lectern and tell your life's story"; "I'll want to drink more after going to a meeting because I've heard that all they talk about is getting high." It is strongly recommended, if you have not done so already, that you attend an AA or NA meeting, and an Al-Anon group, so that you will be able to "poke holes" in your patient's argument about why he or she should not attend a 12 Step meeting. For example, you might inform the patient that, in fact, you have attended a meeting and no one was drunk or high, and no one made anyone stand at a lectern and tell their life's story. You might also suggest that he or she attend the first meeting as an "experiment" to find out firsthand what happens there, and then you can both discuss his or her experience at your next visit. If your patient informs you that he or she went to a meeting but did not feel comfortable there, you might normalize that feeling: "It's normal to feel uncomfortable— you are going to a strange place with people there that you do not know. Everyone feels uncomfortable at their first few meetings. Hang in there and keep going—it will get better. If you *do* continue to feel uncomfortable at that meeting after a few weeks, go ahead and try another AA meeting at a different location."

To paraphrase a statement often said in AA meetings, "No matter how far down the scale we have gone, there is always hope." There are few things as gratifying and moving as watching your addicted patient finally grasp the idea of recovery and begin to blossom in every area of his or her life.

The following points are useful when working with patients who are involved in a 12 Step program, such as AA and NA:

- Ask your patients if they have a *sponsor* (a member of the 12 Step program who has been in the program for an extended period of time and who has completed the 12 Steps). The sponsor functions as a kind of guide and strong support for the newly recovering alcoholic/addict. Encourage your patients who are attending a meeting for the first time to look for someone with whom they relate—someone who seems positive and appears to be doing well in his or her life. Then further encourage your patients to walk up to that person and ask him or her to be a "temporary sponsor" (someone who will function in the sponsor role until your patients find someone else they can better relate to; however, temporary sponsors can become "permanent" sponsors if your patients are happy with the relationship).

- Ask your patients if they are "working the steps." The 12 Steps are completed in a systematic, sequential fashion, with the assistance and guidance of one's sponsor. It is the general feeling in the drug treatment community that members who do not have a sponsor—or are not working on completing the steps—are not really in "recovery" or "sober"; they are merely "abstinent" and may be in a "dry drunk" (e.g., "irritable, restless, discontent"). The 12 Steps are presented in Table 2.1.

- Ask your patients if they have attended "90 meetings in 90 days"—one of the recommendations "old-timers" in the 12 Step programs usually give to "new-comers."

- Ask how many meetings they attend a week and how they feel about going to meetings. Praise patients who are attending meetings regularly, and express your concern to those who are not. One of the many slogans in AA/NA is "meeting makers make it." The converse is also true: it appears that relapse rates are higher for those individuals who do not attend 12 Step meetings regularly.

- Let your patients know that AA and other 12 Step programs are *not* psychotherapy. Consider referral to a therapist who is well-versed in issues surrounding addiction and recovery, in addition to referral to the 12 Step programs.

- Remind your patients to take things *one day at a time*. Patients may feel (understandably) overwhelmed when they think about not drinking or using for the rest of their lives. By breaking sobriety into 24-hour intervals, your patients will find that, after a while, craving will subside and "days sober" or "clean days" will add up. Keep the focus on just today and, if today is difficult, encourage your patients to remember another useful slogan, "this too shall pass."

- Poker chips are given out at the end of each AA and NA meeting to recognize specific numbers of days abstinent. The intervals for these are

Table 2.1. The Twelve Steps of Alcoholics Anonymous.

1. We admitted we were powerless over alcohol; that our lives had become unmanageable.
2. Came to believe that a power greater than ourselves could restore us to sanity.
3. Made a decision to turn our will and our lives over to the care of God *as we understood Him*.
4. Made a searching and fearless moral inventory of ourselves.
5. Admitted to God, to ourselves, and to another human being the exact nature of our wrongs.
6. Were entirely ready to have God remove all these defects of character.
7. Humbly asked Him to remove our shortcomings.
8. Made a list of all persons we had harmed, and became willing to make amends to them all.
9. Made direct amends to such people wherever possible, except when to do so would injure them or others.
10. Continued to take personal inventory and when we were wrong promptly admitted it.
11. Sought through prayer and meditation to improve our conscious contact with God, *as we understood Him*, praying only for knowledge of His will for us and the power to carry that out.
12. Having had a spiritual awakening as the result of these steps, we tried to carry this message to alcoholics, and to practice these principles in all our affairs.

Source: From Alcoholics Anonymous [3], p. 5, with permission of Alcoholics Anonymous World Services, Inc.

usually 30, 60, and 90 days; 6 and 9 months; and year anniversaries. The white chip marks the beginning of the recovery process in the 12 Step programs. A white chip, probably the most important of all, is the first chip your patients will receive (they have to stand up and take the chip at the end of the meeting when the person who is handing out the chips asks, "Is there anyone here who would like a white chip?" This chip signifies the "desire to stop drinking/using . . . just for today." When your patients return for follow-up after their first meeting, ask them if they "got a white chip." If not, encourage them to "pick one up at your next meeting."

- There are no dues or fees in AA/NA, but a basket will be passed around at some point during the meeting for those who would like to donate change or a dollar to help pay for the coffee (which is offered at most meetings) and rent of the meeting space (meetings are usually held in churches, even though the 12 Step programs are not affiliated with any particular religion). Meetings are also held in "meeting rooms" at AA or NA "clubhouses" (buildings, or space in buildings, rented out solely for the purpose of holding 12 Step meetings).
- Alcoholics Anonymous and NA are spiritual, not religious, programs. People from all different religions attend AA and NA meetings, as well as individuals who are not religious but who see themselves as more "spiritual" in their beliefs. These latter individuals may use the term "Higher Power" or other names instead of "God." Atheists and agnostics

also attend the 12 Step programs, but it is strongly believed that all members should develop some type of spiritual understanding in order to maintain abstinence. Throughout the steps, references to the "God of our understanding" can be heard and simply mean that whatever one believes is what works for them. Proselytizing, witnessing, or attempts at converting others to one's own religion are not allowed at 12 Step meetings.

We have included Al-Anon in this section because it is an invaluable resource for the families and friends of the addicted patient (a program called Nar-Anon, affiliated with Narcotics Anonymous, is also available; however, Al-Anon meetings are usually greater in number and are therefore more easily accessible). Al-Anon (and Ala-Teen for the adolescent children of alcoholics) and Nar-Anon teach family members and friends of the alcoholic/addict how to care for themselves and how to avoid, or remove themselves from, the trap of becoming "codependent" (enabling, doing too much for the alcoholic/addict—which ends up hurting that individual, as well as themselves). In addition, these support groups can help the spouse and other family members deal with the major life change that occurs when their loved one finally achieves sobriety/abstinence from all substances. The primary care physician may expect the family to be joyful and supportive when this change occurs; however, the opposite is often true. Family members, who have had their hopes regarding their loved one attaining and maintaining sobriety dashed numerous times over the years, may become anxious, angry and bitter when this change finally does occur. We hypothesize that this latter reaction may be due to a kind of "reality vertigo" (5). Specifically, family members have lived their life with their loved one addicted to a substance for so long that, now that s/he has gotten sober, reality (as they know it) has spun out of control. Even though they will admit that this change is for the better, many family members will report feeling distressed. Many spouses may wonder if this new "drug-free" husband/wife will still love them and/or want to stay in the marriage. Children may feel anxious that the change will not be permanent and that the "rug may be pulled out from under their feet" at any time. Programs such as Al-Anon can help the family to regain balance after this type of reality vertigo due to their loved ones cessation of substance use (5).

The individual who attends these groups will also get a sponsor and start working the steps, but with a different perspective from the alcoholic/addict. Al-Anon and Nar-Anon emphasize that families and friends are "powerless" over (i.e., unable to control) the lives of the alcoholic and addict, whereas AA and NA stress the importance of the alcoholic's and addict's realization of being powerless over alcohol (or one's addiction). Being a primary care physician, you will often treat the entire family, and even the friends, of your alcoholic/addicted patients. It is our recommendation that each of them receives a referral (given to them verbally by you) to attend an Al-Anon meeting. Giving them the phone number to your local Al-Anon office (which, like AA and NA, should be in the White Pages of your phone book), often expedites this process.

It should also be mentioned that even when your addicted patients are in recovery and are no longer actively using substances, they may be engaging in "acting out" behaviors such as gambling, unhealthy sexual behaviors, excessive work, overspending, unhealthy eating, and so on. These behaviors may be an unconscious substitution for the prior substance use and, as mentioned in the previous chapter, they may feed the same neurophysiological reward pathways as did the substances. It is of the utmost importance that you ask your recovering patients about possible acting-out behaviors, because engaging in these may cause patients to relapse into active substance use. If a patient is acting out, suggest that these behaviors are common in recovering individuals and that he or she talk with his or her sponsor and to seek additional help from a counselor/therapist if necessary to work toward a more adaptive way of handling stress.

In summary, in our experience of working with hundreds of patients with substance use disorders throughout the years, the 12 Step programs have proven to be the backbone of long-term recovery—long after detox and subsequent treatment have ended. Again, as is often said in meetings, "meeting makers make it!" Encourage your patients to walk through their (understandable) fear of attending a meeting for the first time and give them hope that they will never have to use substances again . . . one day at a time.

References

1. Alcoholics Anonymous Big Book, 4th ed. New York: Alcoholics Anonymous World Services, Inc.; 2002.
2. Pomm HA, Shahady E, Pomm RM. The CALMER approach: teaching learners six steps to serenity when dealing with difficult patients. Fam Med 2004;36(7):467–469.
3. Alcoholics Anonymous. Twelve Steps and Twelve Traditions. New York: Alcoholics Anonymous World Services, Inc.; 2002.
4. Gold MS (1994). Neurobiology of addiction and recovery: the brain, the drive for the drug, and the 12-step fellowships. J Subst Abuse Treat 1994;11(2):93–97.
5. Pomm HA. Regaining balance after "reality vertigo:" teaching learners to attend to the psychological aspects of patients with chronic, nonmalignant pain. Fam Med 2006; 38:86–89.

3. Clinical Assessment

The primary care physician will see patients who exhibit both covert and overt signs of addiction, often on a regular basis, without ever making the diagnosis of a substance use disorder (SUD). Indeed, research indicates that 9 out of 10 primary care physicians fail to recognize addiction even in patients who present with the classic symptoms of the disease (1). Of course, making this diagnosis is frequently a formidable task in the brief period of time most primary care physicians are afforded in a typical practice. Covert, or hidden, signs of addiction make this difficult task even more daunting. For example, few physicians would suspect that the elderly female patient with a sweet disposition, supportive family, and some trouble with concentration has an SUD. Only by further investigating the cause of her impairment in concentration can the underlying SUD be detected. Overt symptoms, such as obvious intoxication, signs of withdrawal, elevated liver enzymes, and so forth can assist in making the diagnosis of an SUD more readily apparent.

In the interest of parsimony, we focus on office-based clinical indicators of substance use rather than on such indicators as blood alcohol concentration and issues related to driving under the influence of a substance. In addition, we do not discuss assessment of comorbid psychiatric and/or co-occurring substance use disorders in this chapter, although we do touch on these issues in Chapter 4. It is our hope that this chapter gives primary care physicians a variety of tools and information to help them diagnose substance use disorders and recognize the symptoms of withdrawal—even during a 15-minute office visit.

The *Diagnostic and Statistical Manual of Mental Disorders*, fourth edition, text revision (DSM-IV-TR), criteria for substance abuse and substance dependence are presented in Chapter 1 (2). As can be seen from these definitions, a patient diagnosed with substance dependence should not be additionally diagnosed with substance abuse (it is a given that someone who is dependent on a substance is also abusing that substance). This chapter focuses on the recognition of substance abuse, substance dependence, and/or withdrawal symptoms in your clinic patients.

One word of caution pertains to medical records. Once a diagnosis of substance dependence has been given, the patient record, as it relates to this illness, is protected under federal law 42 CFR. In order to release this record, a physician must have a signed release of information on file that complies with this law (please see sample consent form in Chapter 4, Table 4.8).

The Three Cs

One quick and easy way to screen for substance dependence is by educating your patient about the "three Cs." We are uncertain where we first heard of the three Cs; however, one of us (H.P.) has been using this short screen for many years with good results. You might tell your patient that you are concerned about his or her alcohol or other drug use and then ask the patient to think about whether or not he or she answers "yes" to the following:

Because of your (alcohol or other drug use), have you ever had:

- A loss of Control in any area of your life (e.g., forgetting your kid's game, too tired to keep plans with spouse, late for work, etc.)?
- Compulsivity (e.g., using more alcohol or other drug than you intended or for a longer period of time)?
- A time when you kept using despite adverse Consequences (e.g., your family member or friend was worried about your alcohol/other drug use, or you had arguments with loved ones, medical problems, a driving under the influence conviction, or work-related problems, but you kept drinking/using anyway)?

If your patient answers "Yes" to even one of the "Cs," you can let him/her know that s/he may have an alcohol and/or other drug problem that you would like to assess further in order to help him/her.

Behavioral Signs and Symptoms of Addiction (Not All-Inclusive)

If your patients exhibit any of the following signs and symptoms (this list is not all-inclusive), you may want to screen further for the existence of an SUD.

For adults:

- Mood swings
- Personality changes
- Defensiveness—blaming or claiming to be persecuted or victimized
- Conflict with family and/or friends
- Withdrawal from family and friends
- Change in work habits
- Irresponsibility at home and/or work
- Frequent illness
- Poor hygiene
- Apathy, depression, and/or irritability
- Nervousness

For adolescents:

- Change in attitude/personality for no identifiable reason
- Change in friends, new hangouts
- Decreased performance at school, work, and/or home
- Change in activities or hobbies
- Change in habits at home

- Loss of interest in family and family activities
- Forgetfulness and difficulty paying attention
- Lack of motivation, energy, self-esteem—an "I don't care" attitude
- Sudden oversensitivity, temper tantrums
- Moodiness, irritability, or nervousness
- Silliness or giddiness
- Paranoia
- Excessive need for privacy
- Secretive or suspicious behavior
- Chronic dishonesty
- Unexplained need for money
- Change in personal grooming
- Sudden change in wardrobe, hairstyle, or jewelry

The physical examination can also provide clues about the possibility of an underlying SUD. Table 3.1 presents examination findings suggestive of addiction or its complications. As mentioned earlier, many of your patients will present with medical complaints and/or disorders, rather than overt signs of addiction, that are directly related to or caused by their abuse of substances (i.e., medical disorders can be the covert signs of an underlying SUD). Table 3.2 presents selected medical disorders that are related to alcohol or other drug use.

Screening for a Substance Use Disorder by Drug Class: Alcohol

At this time, using laboratory values as a screen for an SUD is most beneficial when the substance of abuse is alcohol. Laboratory markers for other drugs of abuse are not as clear.

Laboratory Values

Mean Corpuscular Volume

An increase in the mean corpuscular volume

- Occurs in approximately one fourth of all alcoholics
- Is often a late sign of alcoholism
- Results from both alcohol's effect on folate metabolism and its direct toxic effect on bone marrow
- Increases with increased alcohol consumption
- Remains elevated for months after cessation of drinking

Gamma-Glutamyl Transpeptidase

The gamma-glutamyl transpeptidase level

Table 3.1. Physical examination findings suggestive of addiction or its complications.

General
- Odor of alcohol on breath
- Odor of marijuana on clothing
- Odor of nicotine or smoke on breath or clothing
- Poor nutritional status
- Poor personal hygiene

Behavior
- Intoxicated behavior during examination
- Slurred speech
- Staggering gait
- Scratching

Skin
- Signs of physical injury
- Bruises
- Lacerations
- Scratches
- Burns
- Needle marks
- Skin abscesses
- Cellulitis
- Jaundice
- Palmar erythema
- Hair loss
- Diaphoresis
- Rash
- Puffy hands

Head, eyes, ears, nose, throat
- Conjunctival irritation or injection
- Inflamed nasal mucosa
- Perforated nasal septum
- Blanched nasal septum
- Sinus tenderness
- Gum disease, gingivitis
- Gingival ulceration
- Rhinitis
- Sinusitis
- Pale mucosae
- Burns in oral cavity

Gastrointestinal
- Hepatomegaly
- Liver tenderness
- Positive stool hemoccult

Immune
- Lymphadenopathy

Cardiovascular
- Hypertension
- Tachycardia
- Cardiac arrhythmia
- Heart murmurs, clicks
- Edema
- Swelling

Pulmonary
- Wheezing, rales, rhonchi
- Cough
- Respiratory depression

Female reproductive/endocrine
- Pelvic tenderness
- Vaginal discharge

Male reproductive/endocrine
- Testicular atrophy
- Penile discharge
- Gynecomastia

Neurologic
- Sensory impairment
- Memory impairment
- Motor impairment
- Ophthalmoplegia
- Myopathy
- Neuropathy
- Tremor
- Cognitive deficits
- Ataxia
- Pupillary dilation or constriction

Source: Adapted from Clinical Guidelines for the Use of Buprenorphine in the Treatment of Opioid Addiction: A Treatment Improvement Protocol (TIP) 40. Rockville, MD: U.S. Department Of Health and Human Services, Substance Abuse and Mental Health Services Administration, Center for Substance Abuse Treatment.

- Increases in approximately two thirds of alcoholics
- Is a sensitive, but not specific, index for alcohol and drug toxicity to the liver (infiltrative liver disorders and/or biliary obstruction)
- Increases after several weeks or longer of heavy alcohol use
- Returns to normal after approximately 3 weeks of abstinence

Table 3.2. Selected medical disorders related to alcohol and other drug use.

Cardiovascular	*Alcohol:* Cardiomyopathy, atrial fibrillation (holiday heart), hypertension, dysrhythmia, masks angina symptoms, coronary artery spasm, myocardial ischemia, high-output states, coronary artery disease, sudden death. *Cocaine:* Hypertension, myocardial infarction, angina, chest pain, supraventricular tachycardia, ventricular dysrhythmias, cardiomyopathy, cardiovascular collapse from body-packing rupture, moyamoya vasculopathy, left ventricular hypertrophy, myocarditis, sudden death, aortic dissection. *Tobacco:* Atherosclerosis, stroke, myocardial infarction, peripheral vascular disease, cor pulmonale, erectile dysfunction, worse control of hypertension, angina, dysrhythmia. *Injection drug use:* Endocarditis, septic thrombophlebitis
Cancer	*Alcohol:* Aerodigestive (lip, oral cavity, tongue, pharynx, larynx, esophagus, stomach, colon), breast, hepatocellular and bile duct cancers. *Tobacco:* Oral cavity, larynx, lung, cervical, esophagus, pancreas, kidney, stomach, bladder. *Injection drug use or high-risk sexual behavior:* Hepatocellular carcinoma related to hepatitis C
Endocrine/ reproductive	*Alcohol:* Hypoglycemia and hyperglycemia, diabetes, ketoacidosis, hypertriglyceridemia, hyperuricemia and gout, testicular atrophy, gynecomastia, hypocalcemia and hypomagnesemia because of reversible hypoparathyroidism, hypercortisolemia, osteopenia, infertility, sexual dysfunction. *Cocaine:* Diabetic ketoacidosis. *Opiates:* Osteopenia, alteration in gonadotropins, decreased sperm motility, menstrual irregularities. *Tobacco:* Graves disease, azoospermia, erectile dysfunction, osteopenia, osteoporosis, fractures, estrogen alterations, insulin resistance. *Any addiction:* Amenorrhea
Hepatic	*Alcohol:* Steatosis (fatty liver), acute and chronic hepatitis (infectious [i.e., B or C] or toxic [i.e., acetaminophen]), alcoholic hepatitis, cirrhosis, portal hypertension and varices, spontaneous bacterial peritonitis. *Cocaine:* Ischemic necrosis, hepatitis. *Opiates:* Granulomatosis. *Injection drug use or high-risk sexual behavior:* Infectious hepatitis B and C (acute and chronic) and delta
Hematologic	*Alcohol:* Macrocytic anemia, pancytopenia because of marrow toxicity and/or splenic sequestration, leukopenia, thrombocytopenia, coagulopathy because of liver disease, iron deficiency, folate deficiency, spur cell anemia, burr cell anemia. *Tobacco:* Hypercoagulability. *Injection drug use or high-risk sexual behavior:* Hematologic consequences of liver disease, hepatitis C–related cryoglobulinemia and purpura
Infectious	*Alcohol:* Hepatitis C, pneumonia, tuberculosis (including meningitis), human immunodeficiency virus (HIV), sexually transmitted diseases, spontaneous bacterial peritonitis, brain abscess, meningitis. *Opiates:* Aspiration pneumonia. *Tobacco:* Bronchitis, pneumonia, upper respiratory tract infections. *Injection drug use:* Endocarditis, cellulitis, pneumonia, septic thrombophlebitis, septic arthritis (unusual joints, i.e., sternoclavicular), osteomyelitis (including vertebral), epidural and

Table 3.2. *Continued*

	brain abscess, mycotic aneurysm, abscesses and soft tissue infections, mediastinitis, malaria, tetanus. *Injection or high-risk sexual behavior:* Hepatitis B, C, and delta; HIV; sexually transmitted diseases
Neurologic	*Alcohol:* Peripheral and autonomic neuropathy, seizure, hepatic encephalopathy, Korsakoff dementia, Wernicke syndrome, cerebellar dysfunction, Marchiafava-Bignami syndrome, central pontine myelinolysis, myopathy, amblyopia, stroke, withdrawal, delirium, hallucinations, toxic leukoencephalopathy, subdural hematoma, intracranial hemorrhage. *Cocaine:* Stroke, seizure, status epilepticus, headache, delirium, depression, hypersomnia, cognitive deficits. *Opiates:* Seizure (overdose and hypoxia), compression neuropathy. *Tobacco:* Stroke, small vessel ischemia, and cognitive deficits. *Any addiction:* Compression neuropathy
Nutritional	*Alcohol:* Vitamin and mineral deficiencies (B_1, B_6, riboflavin, niacin, vitamin D, magnesium, calcium, folate, phosphate, zinc). *Any addiction:* Protein malnutrition
Other gastrointestinal	*Alcohol:* Gastritis, esophagitis, pancreatitis, diarrhea, malabsorption (because of pancreatic exocrine insufficiency, or folate or lactase deficiency), parotid enlargement, malignancy, colitis, Barrett esophagus, gastroesophageal reflux, Mallory-Weiss syndrome, gastrointestinal bleeding. *Cocaine:* Ischemic bowel and colitis. *Opiates:* Constipation, ileus, intestinal pseudo-obstruction. *Tobacco:* Peptic ulcers, gastroesophageal reflux, malignancy (pancreas, stomach). *Any addiction:* Overdose from body-packing.
Prenatal and perinatal	*Alcohol:* Fetal alcohol effects and syndrome. *Cocaine:* Placental abruption, teratogenesis, neonatal irritability. *Opiates:* Neonatal abstinence syndrome, including seizures. *Tobacco:* Teratogenesis, low birth weight, spontaneous abortion, abruptio placentae, placenta previa, perinatal mortality, sudden infant death syndrome, neurodevelopmental impairment.
Perioperative	*Alcohol:* Withdrawal, perioperative complications (delirium, infection, bleeding, pneumonia, delayed wound healing, dysrhythmia), hepatic decompensation, hepatorenal syndrome, death. *Cocaine:* Hypersomnia and depression in withdrawal, mimicking of postoperative neurologic complications, complications from underlying drug-induced cardiopulmonary disease. *Opiates:* Withdrawal, inadequate analgesia. *Tobacco:* Pulmonary infection, difficulty weaning, respiratory failure, reactive airways exacerbations
Pulmonary	*Alcohol:* Aspiration, sleep apnea, respiratory depression, apnea, chemical or infectious pneumonitis. *Cocaine:* Nasal septum perforation, gingival ulceration, perennial rhinitis, sinusitis, hemoptysis, upper airway obstruction, fibrosis, hypersensitivity pneumonitis, epiglottitis, pulmonary hemorrhage, pulmonary hypertension, pulmonary edema, emphysema, interstitial fibrosis, hypersensitivity pneumonia. *Inhalants:* Pulmonary edema,

(Continued)

Table 3.2. *Continued*

	bronchospasm, bronchitis, granulomatosis, airway burns. *Opiates:* Respiratory depression/failure, emphysema, bronchospasm, exacerbation of sleep apnea, pulmonary edema. *Tobacco:* Lung cancer, chronic obstructive pulmonary disease, reactive airways, pneumonia, bronchitis, pulmonary hypertension, interstitial lung disease, pneumothorax. *Injection drug use:* Pulmonary hypertension, talc granulomatosis, septic pulmonary embolism, pneumothorax, emphysema, needle embolization
Renal	*Alcohol:* Hepatorenal syndrome, rhabdomyolysis and acute renal failure, volume depletion and prerenal failure, acidosis, hypokalemia, hypophosphatemia. *Cocaine:* Rhabdomyolysis and acute renal failure, vasculitis, necrotizing angitis, accelerated hypertension, nephrosclerosis, ischemia. *Opiates:* Rhabdomyolysis, acute renal failure, factitious hematuria. *Tobacco:* Renal failure, hypertension. *Injection drug use or high-risk sexual behavior:* Focal glomerular sclerosis (HIV, heroin), glomerulonephritis from hepatitis or endocarditis, chronic renal failure, amyloidosis, nephrotic syndrome (hepatitis C)
Sleep	*Alcohol:* Apnea, periodic limb movements of sleep, insomnia, disrupted sleep, daytime fatigue. *Cocaine:* Hypersomnia in withdrawal. *Opiates:* Insomnia. *Tobacco:* Insomnia, increased sleep latency
Trauma	*Alcohol:* Motor vehicle crash, fatal and nonfatal injury, physical and sexual abuse. *Cocaine:* Death during "Russian roulette." *Opiates:* Motor vehicle crash, other violent injury. *Tobacco:* Burns, smoke inhalation. *Any addiction:* Sexual and physical abuse
Musculoskeletal	*Alcohol:* Rhabdomyolysis, compartment syndromes, gout, saturnine gout, fracture, osteopenia, osteonecrosis. *Cocaine:* Rhabdomyolysis. *Opiates:* Osteopenia. *Any addiction:* Compartment syndromes, fractures

Source: Saitz R. Overview of medical and surgical complications. In Graham AW, Schultz TK, Mayo-Smith MF, Ries RK, Wilford BB, eds. Principles of Addiction Medicine, 3rd ed. Chevy Chase, MD: American Society of Addiction Medicine; 2003. All rights reserved. Reprinted with permission.

Aspartate Aminotransferase and Alanine Aminotransferase

- When the aspartate aminotransferase (AST) level is greater than the alanine aminotransferase (ALT) level, suspect alcoholic hepatitis.
- When the ALT level is increased, check for hepatitis C.

Urine Drug Screens

- Urine drug screens (UDSs) are critical to the assessment process.
- It takes approximately five half-lives for most substances to leave the body (Table 3.3).

Table 3.3. Detection limits of common drugs of abuse in urine drug screens.

Substance	Length of detection
Opiates	
Codeine, morphine, opium	2–4 days
Heroin	2–4 days
Hydromorphine	2–4 days
Meperidine	2–4 days
Methadone	6–12 days
Oxycodone	8–24 hours
Other opiates	8–24 hours
Depressants	
Alcohol	6 hours to 2 days
Barbiturates	2–10 days
Benzodiazepines	1–6 weeks
Methaqualone	2 weeks
Glutethimide	2–10 days
Other depressants	2–7 days
Stimulants	
Cocaine	2–5 days
Amphetamines	1–2 days
Phenmetrazine	1–2 days
Methylphenidate	1–2 days
Nicotine	2–4 days
Other stimulants	1–2 days
Hallucinogens	
LSD	8–24 hours
Mescaline	2–3 days
Amphetamine variants	2–5 days
Phencyclidine	2–4 days
Marijuana	2 days to 11 weeks
THC	2 days to 11 weeks
Hash, hashish oil	2 days to 11 weeks
Other hallucinogens	2–5 days
Steroids	
Nandrolone decanoate	18 months
Nandrolone phenylpropionate	12 months
Boldenone undecylenate	5 months
Methenolone enanthate	
Trenbolone	
Trenbolone acetate	
Injectable methandienone	
Testosterone mix (Sustanon and Omnadren)	3 months

- When at all possible, urine should be collected under observation. If this is not possible, at least have patients leave all items (purses, briefcases, etc.) and outerwear (jackets, bulky sweaters, etc.) outside the room.
- Use a temperature strip to assess the temperature of the urine immediately after it is collected.
- Be certain that laboratories are testing for Xanax, Ativan, Klonopin, and synthetic opioids, as these substances are not necessarily part of a routine urine drug panel.
- Questions regarding false-positive results can often be answered by the laboratory pathologist if a medical review officer has not been part of the validation process. Also remember that a false-positive result for alcohol can occur from in vitro fermentation in the bladder, especially among the diabetic population.
- Investigators have recently been researching the possibility that UDSs can actually be a form of drug treatment/intervention for your patients. In other words, patients may be less likely to use drugs if they know they will be screened on a regular and random basis (3).
- Until recently, because of the rapid metabolism of alcohol, testing for alcohol in the urine was not particularly sensitive. Unless someone had been very recently drinking or had been drinking an excessive amount the night before, a test would often be negative. There is now a urine test for alcohol that is very sensitive and can detect alcohol for up to 80 hours after the complete elimination of alcohol from the body (4). This means that it will detect alcohol for up to 5 days (5) from last consumption. The test is called ethyl glucuronide. Approximately 0.02% of alcohol is metabolized via glucuronidation (6); therefore, it is a direct metabolite. This test allows for the detection of any alcohol consumed, and fermentation is not a factor. However, because of its sensitivity, cut-off levels are very important. In my (R.P.'s) experience, levels between 250 and 500 µg/L should stimulate questions for your patient. Levels above 500 µg/L should be trusted as presumptive of significant alcohol consumption.

Although laboratory values can be helpful tools, clinical interviews and screening instruments are more sensitive and specific for assessing the existence of an underlying SUD.

Screening Instruments: Alcohol Abuse and Dependency

A variety of screening instruments can be used by the primary care physician for the detection of an SUD, and any one instrument is not necessarily better than another. Therefore, it is suggested that you gain a level of comfort with one or two instruments and use them consistently in your practice. The following list is not all-inclusive but does include instruments that the authors believe may be best suited for use in the primary care setting.

The CAGE Questionnaire

The CAGE Questionnaire is quick and reliable and consists of only four questions that you ask your patient (7):

1. Have you ever felt you should **C**ut down on your drinking?
2. Have people **A**nnoyed you by criticizing your drinking?
3. Have you ever felt bad or **G**uilty about your drinking?
4. Have you ever had a drink first thing in the morning to steady your nerves or to get rid of a hangover (**E**ye-opener)?

Scoring: Item responses on the CAGE Questionnaire are scored 0 for "no" and 1 for "yes" answers, with a higher score indicating problems with alcohol. A total score of 2 is clinically significant; however, it is suggested that primary care clinicians lower the threshold to one positive answer to "cast a wider net and identify more patients who may have substance use disorders." (From Ewing JA. Detecting alcoholism. The CAGE questionnaire. JAMA. 1984;252(14):1905–1907. Copyright © 1984, American Medical Association. All rights reserved.)

The Alcohol Use Disorders Identification Test

The Alcohol Use Disorders Identification Test (AUDIT) is another good screening tool (8,9). It consists of 10 questions that, like the CAGE, are asked by the primary care physician. Circle the number that comes closest to the patient's answer:

1. How often do you have a drink containing alcohol?
   (0) Never　　(1) Monthly　　(2) 2–4 times a month
   (3) 2–3 times a week　　(4) 4 or more times a week

2. How many drinks containing alcohol do you have on a typical day when you are drinking? (Code number of "standard" drinks; see definition below.)
   (0) 1–2　　(1) 3–4　　(2) 5–6　　(3) 7–9　　(4) 10 or more

3. How often do you have six or more drinks on occasion?
   (0) Never　　(1) Less than monthly　　(2) Monthly
   (3) Weekly　　(4) Daily or almost daily

4. How often during the last year have you found that you were not able to stop drinking once you had started?
   (0) Never　　(1) Less than monthly　　(2) Monthly
   (3) Weekly　　(4) Daily or almost daily

5. How often during the last year have you failed to do what was normally expected from you because of drinking?
   (0) Never　　(1) Less than monthly　　(2) Monthly
   (3) Weekly　　(4) Daily or almost daily

6. How often during the last year have you needed a first drink in the morning to get yourself going after a heavy drinking session?
   - (0) Never   (1) Less than monthly   (2) Monthly
   - (3) Weekly   (4) Daily or almost daily

7. How often during the last year have you had a feeling of guilt or remorse after drinking?
   - (0) Never   (1) Less than monthly   (2) Monthly
   - (3) Weekly   (4) Daily or almost daily

8. How often during the last year have you been unable to remember what happened the night before because you had been drinking?
   - (0) Never   (1) Less than Monthly   (2) Monthly
   - (3) Weekly   (4) Daily or almost daily

9. Have you or someone else been injured as a result of your drinking?
   - (0) No   (2) Yes, but not in the last year
   - (4) Yes, during the last year

10. Has a relative or friend or a doctor or other health worker been concerned about your drinking or suggested you cut down?
    - (0) No   (2) Yes, but not in the last year
    - (4) Yes, during the last year

One "standard" drink contains 10 g alcohol. In countries where the alcohol content of a standard drink differs by more than 25% from 10 g, the response category should be modified accordingly.

Scoring: Questions 1–8 are scored 0, 1, 2, 3, or 4. Questions 9 and 10 are scored 0, 2, or 4 only. The minimum score (for nondrinkers) is 0, and the maximum score possible is 40. A score of 8 or more indicates a strong likelihood of hazardous or harmful alcohol consumption. (From Babor TF, de la Fuente JR, Saunders J, Grant M. AUDIT: The Alcohol Use Disorders Identification Test: Guidelines for Use in Primary Health Care. Geneva: World Health Organization, 1992.)

Short Michigan Alcohol Screening Test

The Short Michigan Alcohol Screening Test (SMAST) can be used in the primary care setting to assess alcoholism. Ask your patient the following questions, eliciting a "yes" or "no" answer:

1. Do you feel that you are a normal drinker? (By "normal" we mean that you drink less than or as much as most other people.) ___
2. Does your wife, husband, a parent, or other near relative ever worry or complain about you drinking? ___
3. Do you ever feel guilty about your drinking? ___
4. Do friends or relatives think you are a normal drinker? ___

5. Are you able to stop drinking when you want to? ____
6. Have you ever attended a meeting of Alcoholics Anonymous? ____
7. Has drinking ever created problems between you and your wife, husband, a parent, or other near relative? ____
8. Have you ever gotten into trouble at work because of your drinking? ____
9. Have you ever neglected your obligations, your family, or your work for two or more days in a row because you were drinking? ____
10. Have you ever gone to anyone for help about your drinking? ____
11. Have you ever been in a hospital because of drinking? ____
12. Have you ever been arrested for driving under the influence of alcoholic beverages? ____
13. Have you ever been arrested, even for a few hours, because of other drunken behavior? ____

The Short Michigan Alcohol Screening Test is a 13-item questionnaire that requires a 7th grade reading level, and only a few minutes to complete (see next page). It was developed from the Michigan Alcoholism Screening Test. Evaluation data indicate that it is an effective diagnostic instrument, and does not have a tendency for false positives, as does the Michigan Alcoholism Screening Test. Research demonstrates a high degree of reliability with Latino populations, but is useful with all populations.

Administration: Self-administered. All questions are to be answered with "Yes" or "No" answers only.

Scoring: Each "Yes" answer equals one (1) point.

A score of 1 or 2 indicates there is no alcohol problem. A score of 3 indicates a borderline alcohol problem. A score of 4 or more indicates an alcohol problem.

Cost: Since the Short Michigan Alcohol Screening Test is in the public domain, there is no cost for its reproduction and use. Furthermore, as a self-report screening tool, there are no interviewing or administration costs. (From Selzer ML, Vinokur A, van Rooijen L. The Michigan Alcoholism Screening Test and a shortened 13-item version can reliably be used as self-administered questionnaires. Stud Alcohol 1975;36:117–126.)

Skinner Trauma History

The Skinner Scale focuses on trauma that is often related to excessive alcohol use (10). We have found it useful with patients who need more of a backdoor approach (rather than direct questioning about alcohol use at first) because of their level of defensiveness.

Since your 18th birthday, have you . . .

1. Had any fractures/dislocations of bones or joints (excluding sports injuries)?

2. Been injured in a traffic accident?
3. Injured your head (excluding sports injuries)?
4. Been in a fight or assaulted while intoxicated?
5. Been injured while intoxicated?

Scoring: A score of two or more positive responses to the five questions has been shown to indicate a high probability of excessive drinking or alcohol abuse. (From Skinner HA, Holt S, Schuller R, Roy J, Israel Y. Identification of alcohol abuse using laboratory tests and a history of trauma. Ann Intern Med 1984;101(6):847–851.)

Special Populations: Adolescent, Geriatric, and Pregnant Women Alcohol Screening Instruments

Adolescent Alcohol Screen

All adolescents should be asked annually about their use of alcohol, tobacco, and illicit drugs, as well as their use of over-the-counter and prescription drugs for nonmedicinal purposes, including anabolic steroids (11). Urine drug screens should not be used routinely with adolescents; however, they can be a good adjunct to screening questions when there is a reason to suspect drug abuse (11). The CRAFFT scale is a screening tool for adolescents that can be easily incorporated into the medical interview (12):

C: Have you ever ridden in a CAR driven by someone (including yourself) who was "high" or had been using alcohol or drugs?
R: Do you ever use alcohol or drugs to RELAX, feel better about yourself, or fit in?
A: Do you ever use alcohol/drugs while you are by yourself ALONE?
F: Do your FAMILY or FRIENDS ever tell you that you should cut down on your drinking or drug use?
F: Do you ever FORGET things you did while using alcohol or drugs?
T: Have you ever gotten into TROUBLE while you were using alcohol or drugs?

Scoring: A score of two or more positive answers suggests problem use— further assessment/intervention is recommended. (From Knight JR, Shrier LA, Bravender TD, Farrell M, Vander Bilt J, Shaffer HJ. A new brief screen for adolescent substance abuse. Arch Pediatr Adolesc Med 1999;153(6):591–596. Copyright © 1999, American Medical Association. All rights reserved.)

Geriatric Alcohol Screen

The CAGE Questionnaire, with the cut-off score of 1, discussed earlier in this chapter, has been validated as a screening tool with older adults. In addition, the Michigan Alcoholism Screening Test—Geriatric Version (MAST-G) is a valid and reliable measure with this population (13):

1. After drinking, have you ever noticed an increase in your heart rate or beating in your chest?
   YES   NO

2. When talking with others, do you ever underestimate how much you actually drink?
   YES   NO

3. Does alcohol make you sleepy so that you often fall asleep in your chair?
   YES   NO

4. After a few drinks, have you sometimes not eaten or been able to skip a meal because you didn't feel hungry?
   YES   NO

5. Does having a few drinks help decrease your shakiness or tremors?
   YES   NO

6. Does alcohol sometimes make it hard for you to remember parts of the day or night?
   YES   NO

7. Do you have rules for yourself that you won't drink before a certain time of the day?
   YES   NO

8. Have you lost interest in hobbies or activities you used to enjoy?
   YES   NO

9. When you wake up in the morning, do you ever have trouble remembering part of the night before?
   YES   NO

10. Does having a drink help you sleep?
    YES   NO

11. Do you hide your alcohol bottles from family members?
    YES   NO

12. After a social gathering, have you ever felt embarrassed because you drank too much?
    YES   NO

13. Have you ever been concerned that drinking might be harmful to your health?
    YES   NO

14. Do you like to end an evening with a nightcap?
    YES   NO

15. Did you find your drinking increased after someone close to you died?
    YES   NO

16. In general, would you prefer to have a few drinks at home rather than go out to social events?
    YES   NO

17. Are you drinking more now than in the past?
    YES   NO

18. Do you usually take a drink to relax or calm your nerves?
    YES   NO

19. Do you drink to take your mind off your problems?
    YES   NO

20. Have you ever increased your drinking after experiencing a loss in your life?
    YES   NO

21. Do you sometimes drive when you have had too much to drink?
    YES   NO

22. Has a doctor or nurse ever said they were worried or concerned about your drinking?
    YES   NO

23. Have you ever made rules to manage your drinking?
    YES   NO

24. When you feel lonely, does having a drink help?
    YES   NO

Scoring: Five or more "yes" responses are indicative of an alcohol problem. (© The Regents of the University of Michigan, 1991.)

Alcohol Screen for Pregnant Women: The Tweak Test

The TWEAK (Tolerance, Worried, Eye-opener, Amnesia, Kut-down) Test is an effective screening instrument for use with pregnant women (8). In addition, it is suggested that *all pregnant women should be asked, "Do you use street drugs?"* as part of the medical interview. If the patient answers "yes," advise her (and document that you have done so) about the possible negative effects on the fetus and recommend abstinence.

Tolerance: How many drinks can you hold?
Worried: Have close friends or relatives **worried** or complained about your drinking in the past year?
Eye-opener: Do you sometimes take a drink in the morning when you first get up?

Amnesia: Has a friend or family member ever told you about things you said or did while you were drinking that you could not remember?

Kut-down: Do you sometimes feel the need to cut down on your drinking?

Scoring: A 7-point scale is used to score the test. The "tolerance" question scores 2 points if a woman reports she can hold more than five drinks without falling asleep or passing out. A positive response to the "worry" question scores 2 points, and a positive response to the last three questions scores 1 point each. A total score of 3 or 4 usually indicates harmful drinking. For an obstetric patient, a total score of 2 or more indicates the likelihood of harmful drinking. (From Russell M, Czarnecki DM, Cowan R, et al. Measures of maternal alcohol use as predictors of development in early childhood. Alcohol Clin Exp Res 1991;15:991–1000.)

Screening for a Substance Use Disorder by Drug Class: Other Drugs

Many of the previously mentioned screens can be adapted for assessment of other drug use simply by substituting the patient's drug of choice (e.g., cocaine, marijuana, Percocet) for the word "alcohol" and the word "using" instead of "drinking." However, we found several screens that also include the term "other drugs" in their format (14).

The CAGE Questions Adapted to Include Drugs (CAGE-AID)

1. Have you felt you ought to Cut down on your drinking or drug use?
2. Have people Annoyed you by criticizing your drinking or drug use?
3. Have you felt bad or Guilty about your drinking or drug use?
4. Have you ever had a drink or used drugs first thing in the morning to steady your nerves or to get rid of a hangover (Eye-opener)?

Scoring: Item responses on the CAGE-AID are scored 0 for "no" and 1 for "yes" answers, with a higher score indicating problems with alcohol and/or other drugs. A total score of 2 is clinically significant; however, it is suggested that primary care clinicians lower the threshold to one positive answer to "cast a wider net and identify more patients who may have substance use disorders." (From Brown RL, Rounds LA. Conjoint screening questionnaires for alcohol and drug use. WMJ 1995;94:135–140.)

Simple Screening Instrument for Alcohol and Other Drug Use

Another new screen for alcohol and other drug (AOD) use is the Simple Screening Instrument for AOD (15). This tool has not yet been validated, although it shows great promise and should be used with other established screening tools to provide additional information.

Note that **boldface questions** constitute a short version of the screening instrument that can be administered in situations that are not conducive to administering the entire test. Such situations may occur because of time limitations or other conditions.

Use the following introductory statement: "I'm going to ask you a few questions about your use of alcohol and other drugs during the past 6 months. Your answers will be kept private. Based on your answers to these questions, we may advise you to get a more complete assessment. This would be voluntary—it would be your choice whether to have an additional assessment or not. During the past 6 months. . . . "

1. **Have you used alcohol or other drugs? (Such as wine, beer, hard liquor, pot, coke, heroin or other opiates, uppers, downers, hallucinogens, or inhalants.) (yes/no)** (THIS ITEM IS NOT INCLUDED IN THE TOTAL SCORE.)
2. **Have you felt that you use too much alcohol or other drugs? (yes/no)**
3. **Have you tried to cut down or quit drinking or using drugs? (yes/no)**
4. Have you gone to anyone for help because of your drinking or drug use? (Such as Alcoholics Anonymous, Narcotics Anonymous, Cocaine Anonymous, counselors, or a treatment program.) (yes/no)
5. Have you had any of the following? (This item is scored "yes" if any of the items are positive.)
   a. Blackouts or other periods of memory loss
   b. Injury to your head after drinking or using drugs
   c. Convulsions, or delirium tremens ("DTs")
   d. Hepatitis or other liver problems
   e. Feeling sick, shaky, or depressed when you stopped drinking or using drugs
   f. Feeling "coke bugs," or a crawling feeling under the skin, after you stopped using drugs
   g. Injury after drinking or using drugs
   h. Using needles to shoot drugs
6. Has drinking or other drug use caused problems between you and your family or friends? (yes/no)
7. Has your drinking or other drug use caused problems at school or at work? (yes/no)
8. Have you been arrested or had other legal problems? (Such as bouncing bad checks, driving while intoxicated, theft, or drug possession.) (yes/no)

9. Have you lost your temper or gotten into arguments or fights while drinking or using drugs? (yes/no)
10. Are you needing to drink or use drugs more and more to get the effect you want? (yes/no)
11. Do you spend a lot of time thinking about or trying to get alcohol or other drugs? (yes/no)
12. When drinking or using drugs, are you more likely to do something you wouldn't normally do, such as break rules, break the law, sell things that are important to you, or have unprotected sex with someone? (yes/no)
13. Do you feel bad or guilty about your drinking or drug use? (yes/no)
14. Have any of your family members ever had a drinking or drug problem? (yes/no) (THIS ITEM IS NOT INCLUDED IN THE TOTAL SCORE.)
15. **Do you feel that you have a drinking or drug problem now? (yes/no)**
    a. Thanks for answering these questions.
    b. Do you have any questions for me?
    c. Is there something I can do to help you?

Scoring: Questions 1 and 15 are *not* scored. The rest of the items are scored as either 1 (yes) or 0 (no)—the range of scores is 0–14.

Score	Degree of Risk for AOD Abuse
0–1	None to low
2–3	Minimal
≥4	Moderate to high: Possible need for further assessment

Short form: If only the four bold items are used (items 1, 2, 3, 16), a positive answer to any should warrant the administration of the rest of the questions and/or further assessment with another screening tool. (From SAMHSA, TIP 11, Treatment Improvement Protocol (TIP) Series 24. http://www.ncbi.nlm. nih.gov/books.)

Observation checklist: The following signs and symptoms may indicate an AOD abuse problem in the individual being screened:

- Needle track marks
- Skin abscesses, cigarette burns, or nicotine stains
- Tremors (shaking and twitching of hands and eyelids)
- Unclear speech: slurred, incoherent, or too rapid
- Unsteady gait: staggering, off balance
- Dilated (enlarged) or constricted (pinpoint) pupils
- Scratching
- Swollen hands or feet
- Smell of alcohol or marijuana on breath
- Drug paraphernalia such as pipes, paper, needles, or roach clips
- "Nodding out" (dozing or falling asleep)
- Agitation
- Inability to focus
- Burns on the inside of the lips (from freebasing cocaine)

Responding to Positive Screen Results and What to Do Next

If your patient responds positively on a screen and you believe that he or she is abusing alcohol or other drugs, you might say, "After reviewing your answers, there are some things I'd like to follow up with you," or "Your answers to the questions I asked are similar to the answers of people who may be having a problem with alcohol (or other drug)" (6). Three possible approaches are suggested by the Substance Abuse and Mental Health Services Administration based on severity of the problem and possible risk (none of the three is appropriate for an intoxicated patient, who may require an immediate response):

1. The physician can follow up immediately with further questions during the same visit.
2. The physician can schedule a subsequent visit for further questioning if the screening results are inconclusive.
3. The physician can refer after this visit (counseling, Alcoholics or Narcotics Anonymous, etc.; see Chapter 2) while offering ongoing support and encouragement.

As discussed in Chapter 5, it is important to also assess the patient's stage of change (where he or she is with regard to getting help for his or her substance abuse) and then use the appropriate strategy based on that stage.

Assessing Withdrawal Symptoms

Many of your patients may present with withdrawal symptoms. We briefly present withdrawal symptoms for common drugs of abuse; for more detailed diagnostic information, refer to the DSM-IV-TR (2). The management of withdrawal symptoms is discussed in Chapter 4.

Alcohol Withdrawal

- Sleep disturbance
- Gastrointestinal distress (i.e., nausea, vomiting)
- **Diaphoresis**
- Tachycardia
- Transient hallucinations (visual, auditory, tactile), delirium (When your patient presents with one or more of these symptoms, consider this a potential medical emergency and send the patient to the hospital. This

could be delirium tremens, referred to in DSM-IV as alcohol withdrawal delirium.)
- Anxiety
- Tremor
- Agitation
- Seizure

Benzodiazepine Withdrawal

The common signs of benzodiazepine withdrawal are the same as those of alcohol withdrawal, with one exception: no odor of alcohol or of alcoholic metabolites.

Opioid Withdrawal

As discussed in Chapter 4, the symptoms that can commonly develop within minutes to days after cessation include the following:

- Depressed/dysphoric and/or anxious mood
- Gastrointestinal distress (e.g., nausea, vomiting, diarrhea)
- Muscle aches and/or complaints of "bone pain"
- Lacrimation and/or rhinorrhea
- Pupillary dilation
- Piloerection
- Diaphoresis
- Yawning
- Sleep disturbance

Amphetamine Withdrawal

The common symptoms of amphetamine withdrawal include (but may not be limited to) the following:

- Depressed/dysphoric mood
- Hyperphagia
- Hypersomnia or insomnia
- Nightmares
- Fatigue
- Psychomotor agitation or retardation

Nicotine Withdrawal

The common symptoms of nicotine withdrawal, usually manifesting within the first 24 hours, include (but may not be limited to) the following:

- Irritability/anger
- Depressed/dysphoric mood
- Anxiety
- Insomnia
- Increased appetite
- Agitation or restlessness
- Difficulty concentrating and/or sustaining attention
- Mild bradycardia

Instrument for Assessing Withdrawal Symptoms: Alcohol and Benzodiazepines

The Addiction Research Foundation's Clinical Institute Withdrawal Assessment for Alcohol (CIWA-AR) is the most widely used instrument for assessing alcohol and sedative/hypnotic (e.g., benzodiazepine) withdrawal symptoms. The use of this instrument is further detailed in Chapter 4.

Patient:
Date and time:
Pulse or heart rate, taken for 1 minute
Blood pressure:

NAUSEA AND VOMITING—Ask "Do you feel sick to your stomach? Have you vomited?" Observation:
0 No nausea and no vomiting
1 Mild nausea with no vomiting
2
3
4 Intermittent nausea with dry heaves
5
6
7 Constant nausea, frequent dry heaves and vomiting

TACTILE DISTURBANCES—Ask "Have you any itching, pins and needles sensations, any burning, any numbness, or do you feel bugs crawling on or under your skin?" Observation:

0 None
1 Very mild itching, pins and needles, burning, or numbness
2 Mild itching, pins and needles, burning, or numbness
3 Moderate itching, pins and needles, burning, or numbness
4 Moderately severe hallucinations
5 Severe hallucinations
6 Extremely severe hallucinations
7 Continuous hallucinations

TREMOR—Arms extended and fingers spread apart. Observation:
0 No tremor
1 Not visible, but can be felt fingertip to fingertip
2
3
4 Moderate, with patient's arms extended
5
6
7 Severe, even with arms not extended

AUDITORY DISTURBANCES—Ask "Are you more aware of sounds around you? Are they harsh? Do they frighten you? Are you hearing anything that is disturbing to you? Are you hearing things you know are not there?" Observation:
0 Not present
1 Very mild harshness or ability to frighten
2 Mild harshness or ability to frighten
3 Moderate harshness or ability to frighten
4 Moderately severe hallucinations
5 Severe hallucinations
6 Extremely severe hallucinations
7 Continuous hallucinations

PAROXYSMAL SWEATS—Observation:
0 No sweat visible
1 Barely perceptible sweating, palms moist
2
3
4 Beads of sweat obvious on forehead
5
6
7 Drenching sweats

VISUAL DISTURBANCES—Ask "Does the light appear to be too bright? Is its color different? Does it hurt your eyes? Are you seeing anything that is disturbing to you? Are you seeing things you know are not there?" Observation:
0 Not present
1 Very mild sensitivity
2 Mild sensitivity

3 Moderate sensitivity
4 Moderately severe hallucinations
5 Severe hallucinations
6 Extremely severe hallucinations
7 Continuous hallucinations

ANXIETY—Ask "Do you feel nervous?" Observation:
0 No anxiety, at ease
1 Mild anxious
2
3
4 Moderately anxious, or guarded, so anxiety is inferred
5
6
7 Equivalent to acute panic states as seen in severe delirium or acute schizophrenic reactions

HEADACHE, FULLNESS IN HEAD—Ask "Does your head feel different? Does it feel like there is a band around your head?" Do not rate for dizziness or lightheadedness. Otherwise, rate severity:
0 Not present
1 Very mild
2 Mild
3 Moderate
4 Moderately severe
5 Severe
6 Very severe
7 Extremely severe

AGITATION—Observation:
0 Normal activity
1 Somewhat more than normal activity
2
3
4 Moderately fidgety and restless
5
6
7 Paces back and forth during most of the interview or constantly thrashes about

ORIENTATION AND CLOUDING OF SENSORIUM—Ask "What day is this? Where are you? Who am I?" Observation:
0 Oriented and can do serial additions
1 Cannot do serial additions or is uncertain about date
2 Disoriented for date by no more than 2 calendar days
3 Disoriented for date by more than 2 calendar days
4 Disoriented for place/or person

Total CIWA-AR Score_____

Rater's Initials _____

Maximum Possible Score 67

Scoring for the Addiction Research Foundation's Clinical Institute Withdrawal Assessment for Alcohol (CIWA-AR) instrument.

Severity of withdrawal (CIWA-AR score)	Monitoring	Treatment
Mild (≤15)	Assess symptoms with CIWA-AR scale every 4 hours	Thiamine use and supportive care are sufficient if patient has a CIWA-AR score ≤10 and no hallucinations or disorientation. Benzodiazepine therapy may be indicated if score is >10. The goal is a CIWA-AR score below 8 for two consecutive readings
Moderate (16–20)	Assess symptoms with CIWA-AR scale at and 1 hour after each benzodiazepine dose; once score is <10, reassess every 4 hours	Thiamine, supportive care, and benzodiazepine therapy. Benzodiazepine dose every hour, up to three doses, until CIWA-AR score is <10. If no improvement, reassess diagnosis and benzodiazepine dose. Respiratory monitoring advised
Severe (>20)	As for moderate withdrawal	As for moderate withdrawal

Source: From Sullivan JT, Sykora K, Schneiderman J, Naranjo CA, Sellers EM. Assessment of alcohol withdrawal: the revised clinical institute withdrawal assessment for alcohol scale (CIWA-AR). Br J Addict 1989;84(11):1353–1357. Reprinted with permission from Blackwell Publishing.

Instrument for Assessing Withdrawal Symptoms: Opiates

The Clinical Institute Narcotic Assessment Scale measures 11 signs and symptoms commonly seen in patients during narcotic withdrawal. It is presented in Table 3.4. This scale can help to gauge the severity of the symptoms and to monitor changes in the clinical status over time.

Table 3.4. The Clinical Institute Narcotic Assessment (CINA) scale.

Parameters	Findings	Points
Parameters based on questions and observation:		
1. Abdominal changes: Do you have any pains in your abdomen?	No abdominal complaints, normal bowel sounds	0 1 2
	Reports waves of crampy abdominal pain; Crampy abdominal pain, diarrhea, active bowel sounds	
2. Changes in temperature: Do you feel hot or cold?	None reported	0 1 2
	Reports feeling cold, hands cold and clammy to touch	
	Uncontrolled shivering	
3. Nausea and vomiting: Do you feel sick in your stomach? Have you vomited?	No nausea or vomiting	0 2 4 6
	Mild nausea, no retching or vomiting; Intermittent nausea with dry heaves	
	Constant nausea, frequent dry heaves and/or vomiting	
4. Muscle aches: Do you have any muscle cramps?	No muscle aching reported, arm and neck muscles soft at rest	0 1 3
	Mild muscle pains	
	Reports severe muscle pains; muscles in legs, arms, or neck in constant state of contraction	
Parameters based on observation alone:		
5. Goose flesh	None visible	0 1 2 3
	Occasional goose flesh but not elicited by touch; not permanent	
	Prominent goose flesh in waves and elicited by touch	
	Constant goose flesh over face and arms	
6. Nasal congestion	No nasal congestion or sniffling	0 1 2
	Frequent sniffling	
	Constant sniffling, watery discharge	
7. Restlessness	Normal activity	0 1 2 3
	Somewhat more than normal activity; moves legs up and down; shifts position occasionally	
	Moderately fidgety and restless; shifting position frequently	
	Gross movement most of the time or constantly thrashes about	

Table 3.4. *Continued*

Parameters	Findings	Points
8. Tremor	None Not visible but can be felt fingertip to fingertip Moderate with patient's arm extended; Severe even if arms not extended	0 1 2 3
9. Lacrimation	None Eyes watering, tears at corners of eyes; Profuse tearing from eyes over face	0 1 2
10. Sweating	No sweat visible Barely perceptible sweating, palms moist Beads of sweat obvious on forehead Drenching sweats over face and chest	0 1 2 3
11. Yawning	None Frequent yawning Constant uncontrolled yawning	0 1 2
Total score	Sum of points for all 11 parameters	

Note: Minimum score = 0; Maximum score = 31. The higher the score, the more severe the withdrawal syndrome. Percentage of maximal withdrawal symptoms = [(total score)/31] × 100%.
Source: Adapted from Peachey JE, Lei H. Assessment of opioid dependence with naloxone. Br J Addict 1988;83(2):193–201. Reprinted with permission from Blackwell Publishing, Ltd.

References

1. The National Center for Addiction and Substance Abuse (CASA). Missed Opportunity: The CASA National Survey of Primary Care Physicians and Patients 2000. New York: Columbia University. Available at: http://www.casacolumbia.org/absolutenm/templates/PressReleases.aspx?articleid=125&zo.
2. American Psychiatric Association. Diagnostic and Statistical Manual of Mental Disorders, 4th ed, text rev. Washington, DC: American Psychiatric Association; 2000.
3. Jacobs WS, Repetto M, Vinson S, Pomm R, Gold MS. Random urine testing as an intervention for drug addiction. Psychiatric Ann 2004;34(10),781–785.
4. Wurst FM, Skipper GE, Weinmann W. Ethyl glucuronide—the direct ethanol metabolite on the threshold from science to routine use. Addiction 2003;98:51–61.
5. Skipper GE, Weinmann W, Thierauf A, Schaefer P, Wiesbeck G, Allen JP, Miller M, Wurst FM. Ethyl glucuronide: a biomarker to identify alcohol use by health professionals recovering from substance use disorders. Alcohol Alcohol 2004;39(5):445–449.

6. Goll M, Schmitt G, Ganssmann B, Aderjan RE. Excretion profiles of ethyl glucuronide in human urine after internal dilution. J Anal Toxicol 2002;26:262–266.

7. Ewing JA. Detecting alcoholism. The CAGE questionnaire. JAMA 1984;252(14): 1905–1907.

8. Babor TF, de la Fuente JR, Saunders J, Grant M. AUDIT: The Alcohol Use Disorders Identification Test: Guidelines for Use in Primary Health Care. Geneva: World Health Organization; 1992.

9. Sullivan E, Fleming M, co-chairs. A Guide to Substance Abuse Services for Primary Care Clinicians. Treatment Improvement Protocol (TIP) Series 24. Rockville, MD: Substance Abuse and Mental Health Services Administration, U.S. DHHS; 1997. Available at: http://www.ncbi.nlm.nih.gov/books/bv.fcgi?rid=hstat5.chapter.45293.

10. Skinner HA, Holt S, Schuller R, Roy J, Israel Y. Identification of alcohol abuse using laboratory tests and a history of trauma. Ann Intern Med 1984;101(6):847–851.

11. American Medical Association. Guidelines for Adolescent Preventative Services (GAPS) Recommendations Monograph. Chicago: Department of Adolescent Health, American Medical Association; 1997.

12. Knight JR, Shrier LA, Bravender TD, Farrell M, Vander Bilt J, Shaffer HJ. A new brief screen for adolescent substance abuse. Arch Pediatr Adolesc Med 1999;153(6): 591–596.

13. Blow FC, Brower KJ, Schulenberg JE, Demo-Dananberg LM, Young JP, Beresford TP. The Michigan Alcoholism Screening Test—Geriatric Version (MAST-G): a new elderly-specific screening instrument. Alcohol Clin Exp Res 1992;16:372.

14. Brown RL, Rounds LA. Conjoint screening questionnaires for alcohol and drug use. WMJ 1995;94:135–140.

15. Winters KC, Zenilman JM, co-chairs. Simple Screening Instruments for Outreach for Alcohol and Other Drug Abuse and Infectious Diseases. Treatment Improvement Protocol (TIP) Series 11. Rockville, MD: Substance Abuse and Mental Health Services Administration, U.S. DHHS; 1995. Available at: http://www.ncbi.nlm.nih.gov/books.

4. Pharmacologic Office-Based Interventions

Most, if not all, primary care physicians will be faced with the question of how to manage the addicted/alcoholic patient. In this chapter, we discuss how to (1) determine when you should utilize inpatient versus outpatient detoxification; (2) become knowledgeable regarding various methods of outpatient detoxification for each of the specific drugs of abuse; (3) manage patients pharmacologically after discharge from an inpatient detoxification setting; and (4) use the various medications available for your patients to assist in minimizing their relapse potential.

The first, and maybe most important, concept is that *detoxification is not treatment* (1). Detoxification (from this point on we use the terms *detox* or *detoxing* interchangeably) is only a means by which one can more safely and comfortably experience the reduction of the more harmful levels of the addictive substance(s) in the body. This process does not reverse the longer term changes the drug(s) has caused in the body's neurophysiologic response, but it does allow the body to begin this reversal without putting the patient at risk for a potentially life-threatening acute withdrawal reaction. Also, eliminating the drug(s) from the body allows your patients the best possible opportunity to begin the process of learning about this disease and to acquire the "tools" necessary to begin, as well as maintain, their lifelong journey of recovery.

The two treatment milieu alternatives for detox are outpatient and inpatient. Determining which setting is the safest and most beneficial for your patients can be complicated and is explained in some detail as each substance is discussed (Table 4.1). Some of the general concepts concerning the indications for outpatient detox are as follows:

- A life-threatening situation does not exist. Outpatient detox is not appropriate for pregnant women; they need inpatient detox with fetal monitoring available.
- The patient must be able to fully understand the protocol being used and the potential signs and symptoms that he or she might experience during the detox process.
- The patient must be educated about and express an understanding of the risks and benefits of inpatient versus outpatient detox.
- The patient should live with, or at least have ready access to, a stable, positive support system (family, significant other, etc.). The support person(s) should stay with your patient during the most critical time periods of the protocols as well as be able to drive your patient to and from the first several appointments.
- Preferably, the patient should have a stable income.

Table 4.1. Summary of inpatient versus outpatient treatment indicators.

Indicator	Outpatient/inpatient
Clinical Institute Withdrawal Assessment score <15	+/−
Non-life threatening	+/−
No history of acute withdrawal seizures or delirium	+/−
Able to comply with treatment plan	+/−
Potential serious psychiatric comorbidity	−/+
Positive social/financial support	+/−
Appropriate stage of change (i.e., Preparation or Action)	+/−

+, Positive indicator; −, negative indicator.

- The patient should be in the appropriate stage of change (i.e., Preparation or Action; see Chapter 5) and be very motivated to stop using substances.
- The patient should not have a potentially serious and/or unstable comorbid psychiatric and/or medical condition.
- When possible, the supportive family member or significant other should attend an appointment prior to beginning the process during which you can educate him or her regarding the protocol, as well as the signs, symptoms, and potential complications that require a phone call to your office or a call to 911. This informational meeting can save you from many phone calls and the patient from much unnecessary worry.
- You or your nurse should be initially available for frequent appointments.
- Document everything you have done in preparation for the detox procedure or reasons for referral to an inpatient milieu.

Assuming that all the above points have been appropriately addressed, we are now ready to discuss some specific protocols and details for each of the more popular drugs classes that are being abused.

Alcohol: Basics and Detoxification

Before discussing the various detox protocols for alcohol, we present some important concepts specific to alcohol that must be understood:

- A significant amount of alcohol, as previously mentioned, is absorbed by the stomach (about 25%), small intestine, and colon.
- Food can interfere with its absorption, and it is primarily metabolized by the liver.
- The odor of alcohol on the breath is not indicative of the amount of alcohol consumed due to the odor being only representative of the impurities.

- The rate that alcohol is metabolized is constant and is determined by zero order kinetics (a constant amount is metabolized per unit of time). In fact, alcohol is the only drug to be discussed in this book that operates according to this pharmacokinetic process.
- A 1.5-ounce shot of 80 proof alcohol is equal to a 12-ounce can of beer and also to 5 ounces of wine.
- It takes approximately 1 to 1.5 hours for the body to metabolize the equivalent of 1–1.5 oz of an 80–100 proof shot of alcohol. In this regard, the blood alcohol content (BAC) of an individual drops approximately 15–20 mg/dL per hour (0.015–0.020 mg % per hour).

Now let us look at the effect of the BAC on the individual. Obviously, the higher the BAC, the more impaired the individual (Table 4.2).

- An individual under the influence of alcohol cannot be assumed to have the requisite ability to give informed consent.
- If your patient is intoxicated at the office visit and the protocol has previously been discussed with your patient and the support person, an emergency room visit would be in order, and the protocol can be started by the emergency room physician, in communication with you, once the BAC is ≤150 mg/dL, to be followed up by you the next day.
- You should anticipate potential severe withdrawal and refer for inpatient detox if the BAC is >200 mg/dL and the patient is *not* showing signs of intoxication. Common signs of alcohol intoxication include (but are not limited to) the following:
  ○ Impairments in memory, attention and/or concentration
  ○ Unsteady gait
  ○ Slurred speech
  ○ Incoordination
  ○ Stupor or coma

Table 4.2. Concentration–effect relationship of alcohol.

Blood alcohol concentration (%)	Effects
0.02–0.03	Mood elevation. Slight muscle relaxation
0.05–0.06	Relaxation and warmth. Increased reaction time. Decreased fine muscle coordination
0.08–0.09	Impaired balance, speech, vision, hearing, muscle coordination. Euphoria
0.14–0.15	Gross impairment of physical and mental control
0.20–0.30	Severely intoxicated. Very little control of mind or body
0.40–0.50	Unconscious. Deep coma. Death from respiratory depression

Source: Courtesy of Alcohol Use and its Medical Consequences, Project Cork of Dartmouth Medical School, 1981; and Alcohol Medical Scholars Program. With permission.

- A urine drug screen (UDS) is mandatory before the detox protocol is begun, because the presence of multiple substances might preclude the use of an outpatient modality and will certainly alter your management of the situation.

One last important point to consider prior to making the decision for outpatient detox is whether your patient has a history of any of the following serious medical conditions. If your patient has a history of alcohol withdrawal-related seizures or alcohol withdrawal delirium, previously known as *delirium tremens* (see the *Diagnostic and Statistical Manual of Mental Disorders*, fourth edition, text revision [DSM-IV-TR]; considered to be a medical emergency), his or her chances of having the same recur during a subsequent attempt at withdrawal is very likely. In fact, related to alcohol-induced seizures, a kindling effect occurs, which translates into the seizures becoming more severe with each subsequent withdrawal episode (2). Therefore, we would not recommend the use of an outpatient setting for such a patient. However, for those patients without this type of history, in one author's (R.P.'s) experience, utilizing the protocols soon to be described, he has never seen a patient have an alcohol withdrawal seizure unless the detox was started too late. The diagram in Figure 4.1 gives an approximate time frame of when either of these two conditions might be expected to occur.

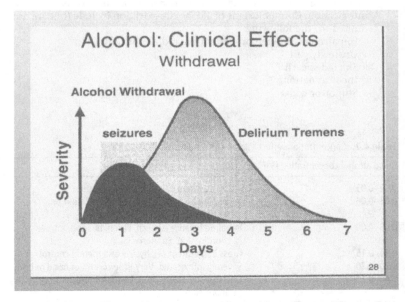

Figure 4.1. Clinical effects of alcohol withdrawal. (From Koch-Weser J, Sellers EM, Kalant H. Alcohol intoxication and withdrawal. N Engl J Med 1976;294:757–762. Copyright ©1976 Massachusetts Medical Society. All rights reserved. Reprinted with permission.)

To help prevent the onset of either alcohol withdrawal-related seizures or alcohol withdrawal delirium, the patient should have an adequate blood level of benzodiazepine prior to day 2. If you utilize the Clinical Institute Withdrawal Assessment (CIWA-AR; see Chapter 3) instrument and his or her score is not above 10 on initial assessment, you might have the patient sit in your office waiting room for several hours. Of course he or she can come and go but should return to the office upon development of any further or worsening symptoms. If your patient has a CIWA-AR score between 10 and 15, and an outpatient detox program has been agreed on, you can initiate the treatment protocol. If the score is over 15, you must make a decision based on your comfort level as to which setting is going to be safest, realizing that the greater the score, the more severe the withdrawal. Not using the CIWA-AR (or the equivalent) is permissible, but you will have to start the protocol as soon as your patient arrives at your office, as predetermined by your agreement with the patient.

Librium (chlordiazepoxide) is still the mainstay of alcohol detoxification. One benefit of this drug is its long half-life, of up to 200 hours (including its active metabolites), which translates into it being self-weaning. The protocol allows for an adequate (not excessive) increase followed by a slow decrease in blood level (considering a normally functioning liver in a relatively healthy, nongeriatric patient).

The basic Librium protocol is as follows:

- 25–50 mg four times per day for 2 days
- 25–50 mg three times per day for 2 days
- 25–50 mg two times per day for 2 days
- 25–50 mg one time per day for 2 days and then discontinue

If you are concerned about potentially mild levels of hepatic compromise (elevated liver enzymes, but otherwise asymptomatic) or interaction with other medications or your patient is geriatric, you can substitute Ativan (lorazepam) 1.0–2.0 mg (higher dosing is utilized in an inpatient setting) in the above protocol. If the level of hepatic compromise is more than mild, you should refer for inpatient detox.

Generally speaking, your patient should have adequate nutritional support and be taking a multivitamin in addition to a good B-complex vitamin that includes 100 mg of thiamine. Also, schedule daily visits with you or your nurse to check vital signs and CIWA-AR score to ensure that the patient is following the protocol and adequately responding; therefore, starting the protocol on a Monday is preferable when possible.

If your patient has returned to see you after completion of an inpatient detoxification program but is still uncomfortable, you can start the outpatient protocol at any point you feel it is indicated. The closer the patient's CIWA-AR score is to 15, the more likely you should start at the beginning. Remember two things: (1) the more comfortable your patient is, the more likely he or she will be amenable to and capable of continuing to learn about and attain long-term abstinence; (2) your patient's urine will more than likely test positive for benzodiazepines and/or barbiturates, depending on what was utilized for the inpatient detox protocol, so do not assume new use of this substance. In addition, try to obtain a release of information to talk with the inpatient provider before initiating any further treatment (releases are mandatory for drug and alcohol treatment facilities, as this is a federal requirement under CFR42).

Finally, if you are concerned about possible drug seeking or that your patient might abuse your protocol medication, we recommend that he or she be given a new prescription for the following 24 hours' worth of medication each visit. When utilizing this approach, be certain that your patient uses only one pharmacy during this process and that you discuss your treatment plan with the pharmacist beforehand. For more information on alcohol dependence, see the references listed here (3,4).

Anxiolytics/Hypnotics: Basics and Detoxification

The focus of our discussion as it relates to this class of drug is on the benzodiazepines. The most likely abused barbiturate is butalbital (i.e., Fioricet and Fiorinal), and, when this is of concern, we would recommend referral for inpatient detoxification. Barbiturates, although not commonly abused compared with other drugs in this class, can have far greater associated risks than benzodiazepines during the detox process.

Benzodiazepines are, in many ways, similar to alcohol (although they appear to bind primarily to the gamma-aminobutyric acid [GABA] receptor as compared with the more diverse utilization of receptors by alcohol). In fact, benzodiazepines are, in some circles, called "dry alcohol." In this regard, the common signs of benzodiazepine intoxication are the same as those of alcohol intoxication with one exception: no odor of alcohol.

The CIWA-AR or a similar withdrawal scale, as discussed with alcohol, can also be used in the assessment of benzodiazepine withdrawal. Also, as with alcohol, a prior history of withdrawal seizures (kindling effect) and/or withdrawal delirium should be considered a contraindication for outpatient detox. Even a prior history of these withdrawal difficulties with alcohol (and no prior history with benzodiazepines) would still bear the same weight for decisions regarding the detox setting for benzodiazepines because of crossover between the two substances.

One significant difference compared with alcohol that must be considered with benzodiazepines is the concept of half-life. This parameter is critical in assessing withdrawal symptoms and symptom risk. Therefore, let us first review the half-life information for some of the more commonly used benzodiazepines (Table 4.3).

When assessing withdrawal symptoms, as previously stated, one may use the CIWA-AR, but, secondary to the half-life, symptoms may not appear shortly after cessation of use (as one would see with alcohol). The most critical period of time for the shorter half-life drugs (i.e., Xanax and Ativan) is 2–4 days after cessation. However, the most critical period of time for the longer half-life drugs (i.e., Valium and Klonopin) is 6–8 days after cessation. However, when abuse has been confirmed, we would still recommend starting the detox protocol as soon after cessation as possible, even though the CIWA-AR score might be low. Waiting for symptoms to develop, depending on half-life and time from cessation, might place the patient at a greater risk for seizures.

Before we look at the actual protocols, further discussion regarding the problems associated with the use and abuse of benzodiazepines is warranted. Xanax (alprazolam) is probably the most commonly prescribed and most commonly abused benzodiazepine. In the authors' as well as many other professionals' opinion, it has the most complicated therapeutic and withdrawal picture compared to other drugs in this class. Secondary to its rapid onset of action and relatively short half-life, its addiction potential is greater than that of many other benzodiazepines. In fact, even at therapeutic dosing levels, tolerance and withdrawal developed more rapidly (4 days for tolerance and 2 days for withdrawal) than was the case with lorazepam and Klonopin (clonazepam) (7 days for tolerance; 4 days for withdrawal) (5–7). Also, interdose withdrawal is particularly problematic with this medication, especially because the symptoms during the interdose phase can be virtually indistinguishable from the very symptoms that prompted treatment in the first place (withdrawal or symptom reemergence?). Last, but not least, alprazolam withdrawal can be very difficult. In fact, in one author's (R.P.'s) experience, many addicts often report that this particular withdrawal was the worst they had ever experienced. However, we will discuss ways in which you can gain the tools needed to successfully detox your motivated patients from this type of medication.

Other general concepts regarding the use and withdrawal of benzodiazepines need to be mentioned. High-dose (two to three times the upper limit of recommended therapeutic dosing) withdrawal is best left for the inpatient setting. However, given the motivated, reliable patient, low-dose (therapeutic dosing, even at high or a little higher than the upper recommended limits of short term or chronic use) withdrawal can and often should be handled on an outpatient basis.

Some of the nonbenzodiazepine sedative hypnotic drugs, such as zaleplon (Sonata), zolpidem (Ambien), and eszopiclone (Lunesta), are addictive and can be abused. These drugs still bind to the same receptors and can cause withdrawal difficulties after long-term use or abuse. In addition, carisoprodol (Soma), often used as a muscle relaxant, is often abused, especially with opioids. This particular drug is problematic as it metabolizes to meprobamate, which can present a more complicated barbiturate-like withdrawal picture. In fact, we highly recommend staying away from prescribing any of these medications to patients who have an abuse/dependence history or potential problem.

We now look at three different types of withdrawal protocols. If your patient is dependent on long half-life benzodiazepines, such as Valium (diazepam), you can use the same drug for detox purposes. If your patient is dependent on shorter half-life medications, such as lorazepam or Serax (oxazepam), you can still use the same drug for detox purposes. However, R.P. and many of his colleagues have rarely been able to successfully detox a patient from alprazolam by using alprazolam. The peaks and valleys associated with the short half-life and rapid onset of action along with the interdose withdrawal problems make this type of detox uncomfortable for the patient and therefore compliance is unlikely. In the case of alprazolam, the author recommends substituting Klonopin (clonazepam) at a ratio of 1–1.5 mg (only rarely 1.5 mg

Table 4.3. Pharmacokinetic properties of benzodiazepines.

Generic name (brand name)	Dosage equivalent (mg)	Onset of action	Relative lipophilicity	Active substances	Elimination half-life (hr)*	Metabolism
Clonazepam (Klonopin)	0.25	Intermediate	+½	Clonazepam	18–50	Oxidation Nitroreduction
Alprazolam (Xanax)	0.5	Intermediate	+++	Alprazolam	6–20	Oxidation
				Alpha-hydroxyalprazolam	6–10	
Triazolam (Halcion)	0.5	Fast	+++	Triazolam	1.7–3.0	Oxidation
Lorazepam (Ativan)	1.0	Intermediate	++½	Lorazepam	10–20	Conjugation
Estazolam (ProSom)	2	Intermediate	++	Estazolam	8–24	Oxidation
Diazepam (Valium and others)	5.0	Fast	+++++	Diazepam	30–100	Oxidation
Clorazepate† (Tranxene)	7.5	Fast	++++	Desmethyldiazepam	30–200	Oxidation
				Oxazepam	3–11	
Chlordiazepoxide (Librium and others)	10.0	Intermediate	++½	Chlordiazepoxide	5–100	Oxidation

Drug (brand)	Dose	Onset	Potency	Active metabolite (elimination, h)	Metabolism
				Desmethylchlordiazepoxide 18	
				Demoxepam 14–95	
				Desmethyldiazepam 30–200	
Oxazepam (Serax)	15.0	Slow	++	Oxazepam 3–21	Conjugation
Flurazepam (Dalmane)	30.0	Fast		Flurazepam 05–3.5	Oxidation
				Hydroxyethylflurazepam 1–4	
				Desalkylflurazepam 48–120	
Temazepam (Restoril)	30.0	Slow	+++	None 10–12	Conjugation
Quazepam (Doral)	30	Fast	+++++	Quazepam 20–120	Oxidation
				Oxoquazepam	
				Desalkylflurazepam‡	
Buspirone (Buspar)	15–30 (usual dose)	Rapid peak, very slow onset (>7 days)		1-Pyrimidinyl piperazine 2–11	
Zolpidem (Ambien)	10	Rapid		Zolpidem 2.5	

* Elimination represents the total for all active metabolites.

† Clorazepate is a prodrug that is converted in the stomach to desmethyldiazepam, the active substance in the blood.

‡ Desalkylflurazepam is identical to N-desalkyl-2-oxoquozepam.

Source: Graham AW, Schultz TKP. Principles of Addiction Medicine, 2nd ed. Bethesda, MD: American Society of Addiction Medicine; 1998, with permission; adapted from Cowley OS, Roy-Byrne PP, Greenblatt DL. Benzodiazepines: pharmacokinetics and pharmacodynamics. In Roy-Byrne PP, Cowley DS, eds. Benzodiazepines in Clinical Practice: Risks and Benefits. Washington, DC: American Psychiatric Press; 1991;26–27 (with permission).

is needed, usually starting at a 1 mg : 1 mg ratio is adequate) clonazepam for every milligram of alprazolam (the higher the dose of alprazolam, the lower end of the ratio to be used). Clonazepam tends to be smoother (without the peaks and valleys), have a slower onset of action and longer half-life, and no active metabolites. Therefore, this drug tends to be self-weaning.

No matter which drug you choose to use for your detox protocol, it should be given in divided doses, either three time per day (tid) or four times per day (qid). For the patient who is chemically dependent (an addict), we recommend a faster rather than slower weaning at a rate not faster than 10% of the original abused (or equivalent) amount per day reduction until discontinuation (i.e., if diazepam is being abused at a dose of 100 mg/day, you would reduce the total daily amount given in divided doses no quicker than 10 mg/day). Although not necessary, it is often easier for the patient, on, for example, a qid schedule to reduce in this order: each dose via a rotational schedule with the 12 noon dose first, 4 pm second, morning (am) third, and the bedtime (hs) last. Decreasing the bedtime dose last in each rotational cycle is most desirable as this is the longest period of time in a 24-hour period during which the patient will be between doses. Table 4.4 shows an example using diazepam (one can substitute any benzodiazepine in this protocol).

Ten percent reduction per day is the fastest approach that can safely be taken. At times, one might have to hold up the reduction or back it up one step for a day or more to allow for restabilization. A motivated, reliable patient who is not an addict/alcoholic and is on a low-dose, long-term therapeutic dosing schedule whom you wish to wean can and probably should be detoxed much more slowly, that is, over the course of 1 or more months. Keeping these patients as comfortable as possible can improve the outcome.

Table 4.4. Sample detoxification protocol for diazepam.

Day	Morning	Noon	4 pm	Bedtime
1	25	25	25	25
Continue for 1–2 days to stabilize at qid dosing schedule				
3	25	15	25	25
4	25	15 mg	15	25
5	15	15	15	25
6	15 qid			
7	15	5	15	15
8	15	5	5	15
9	5	5	5	15
10	5 qid			
11	5	0	5	5
12	5	0	0	5
13	0	0	0	5
14	Discontinue			

Note: All dosages are in milligrams. qid, four times a day.

As with the alcoholic whom you suspect might abuse your prescriptions over the shorter detox schedule, we strongly suggest you institute daily visits and daily prescriptions as described in the section on alcohol detox. These visits can be managed by you or your nurse.

In addition, for those patients taking benzodiazepines as a treatment for an anxiety disorder (without a concomitant addiction problem), consider adding a selective serotonin reuptake inhibitor antidepressant prior to beginning your protocol, as these medications can be a very effective treatment choice for anxiety disorders (without the complications of addictive medications). Be certain the patients are tolerating a therapeutic dose of a selective serotonin reuptake inhibitor for 1 to 2 weeks prior to beginning the dose reduction. If, along the way, your patient experiences symptoms that you are not sure are caused by withdrawal or symptom reemergence, remember, you can back up a step or two and restabilize prior to restarting the protocol from that new set point. Slow is good for this type of patient, while allowing for the possibility of many stops and steps back with restabilization along the way. Progress and patient compliance are paramount.

For this type of schedule (as delineated in the prior paragraph), initial weekly visits and helping the patient feel that he or she is in control of the withdrawal schedule through communication with you is very important. Remember, the patient is not going to be totally symptom free through this process and will need much encouragement. Eventually, scheduling of visits can become more flexible, based on need.

Opioids: Basics and Detoxification

We will review a few basics before we discuss the detoxification protocol for opioids.

- For the purpose of this book, the primary receptor to which opioids bind is the mu receptor.
- There are at least two other receptors, kappa and delta, but the mu receptor is the most responsible for the analgesia and euphoria (also miosis, constipation, and respiratory depression).
- Opioids, as a class of drugs, can be broken down into agonists and partial agonists. In addition, we will discuss opioid antagonists (Table 4.5).
- Agonists bind to the receptor and activate it. Partial agonists bind to the receptor and partially activate it. Antagonists bind to the receptor and inhibit it.
- If you give a mixed agonist–antagonist to an opiate addict, you will precipitate an acute withdrawal (as the antagonist displaces the agonist from the receptor). This is similar to administering naloxone (only available in subcutaneous, intramuscular, and intravenous forms, with action lasting minutes) or naltrexone (available orally and recently in a monthly intramuscular injection, with action lasting hours). Therefore, stay away from prescribing these types of drugs to addicts (except Narcan in overdose situations and naltrexone for opiate addicts who are abstinent

Table 4.5. Agonist, partial agonist, and antagonist opioids.

Agonists
    Codeine
    Fentanyl
    Heroin
    Hydrocodone (Tussionex)
    Hydromorphone (Dilaudid)
    Morphine
    Methadone
    Meperidine (Demerol)
    Oxycodone (Percodan and OxyContin)
    Propoxyphene (Darvon, Darvocet)
Partial agonists
    Buprenorphine (Buprenex, Subutex, Suboxone)
Mixed agonist–antagonists
    Butorphanol (Stadol)
    Nalbuphine (Nubain)
    Pentazocine (Talwin)
Antagonists
    Naloxone (Narcan)
    Naltrexone (Trexan)

and fit into the patient population in which it has been shown to help maintain abstinence—to be discussed later).

- In a somewhat different way, if you give buprenorphine to an opiate addict and the level of opioid being consumed is greater than that being given in the form of buprenorphine, acute withdrawal will also be precipitated. Buprenorphine binds very tightly to the receptor and basically displaces the other agonists, but it only partially activates the receptor, that is, a partial agonist, therefore bringing the opioid level of activity only partially up to the level to which the addict has become tolerant.
- Tolerance to the euphorigenic effects of opioids builds fairly rapidly with regular use (there is minimal tolerance to the constipation or miosis). Interestingly, especially with the longer half-life opioids, tolerance to the analgesic effects is also minimal.
- OxyContin is oxycodone within a vehicle that allows slow release. Therefore, the dose of oxycodone in OxyContin is far greater than that of Percodan or Percocet. However, addicts quickly learn that if they compromise the vehicle (scratching the surface off or crushing the tablet), they can swallow, insufflate, or deliver intravenously a large bolus of oxycodone. Unfortunately, their tolerance might not be at the level that allows such a large dose, and they can die.
- Alcohol and/or benzodiazepines taken with opiates increase the respiratory depressant effect of any one of these drugs individually.

Common signs of opioid intoxication include the following:

- Pupillary constriction
- Impairment in attention/memory/concentration
- Drowsiness or coma
- Slurred speech (often not as pronounced as one might find with alcohol intoxication)

Unfortunately, in one author's (R.P.'s) experience, except when an addict is under the initial acute effects of opioids (even heroin), it is difficult to recognize when a patient is under the influence of this category of drug. Pupillary constriction in a dimly lit room can be of benefit in this regard. A positive UDS result is often the only firm evidence you may have at the time (see Chapter 3 for complete details on UDSs).

With regard to opioid withdrawal, it is important to know a few facts. Some of the symptoms that can commonly develop within minutes to days after cessation include the following:

- Depressed, dysphoric, and/or anxious mood
- Gastrointestinal distress (i.e., nausea, vomiting, and/or diarrhea)
- Muscle aches and/or complaints of "bone pain"
- Lacrimation and/or rhinorrhea
- Pupillary dilation
- Piloerection
- Diaphoresis
- Yawning
- Sleep disturbance

Fortunately, opioid withdrawal does not typically lead to death, although addicts might feel as if they are dying. Therefore, some of the cautions noted in the sections on alcohol and benzodiazepines are not necessary here. However, by the time opioid addicts want detox, they are receiving very little euphoria compared with the far greater amount of time spent attempting to attenuate the withdrawal symptoms by continued use. In this regard, for our purposes, for the remainder of this topic, the Clinical Institute Narcotic Assessment Scale (see Chapter 3) or the Clinical Opiate Withdrawal Scale (not discussed in this book) can be helpful in assessing the severity of withdrawal symptoms.

Another important fact has to do with the identification of the role of the locus coeruleus in withdrawal. The locus coeruleus is located in the dorsolateral pontine tegmentum. It contains the largest grouping of norepinephrine-containing neurons in the brain (8). When one takes opioids, the release of norepinephrine is inhibited (a desired effect is postmyocardial infarction). During withdrawal, greater than normal amounts of norepinephrine are released, and this is underlying many of the major withdrawal symptoms; therefore, the main detox protocol centers on this concept.

Basic to this protocol is the alpha-2 agonist clonidine. This particular drug is very effective in the management of the norepinephrine-based symptoms (9,10). Usual doses are 0.1–0.2 mg every 3–6 hours as needed for withdrawal symptoms, not to exceed 1.2 mg per day as an outpatient. Be sure to monitor blood pressure 1 hour after the first dose and daily as indicated. After 1 to 2

Table 4.6. Clonidine patch protocol.

Weight	Week 1	Week 2	Week 3	Week 4	Week 5
<110 lbs	1 TTS-2	1 TTS-1	None	None	None
110–160 lbs	1 TTS-3	1 TTS-2	1 TTS-1	None	None
160–200 lbs	2 TTS-2	1 TTS-3	1 TTS-2	1 TTS-1	None
>200 lbs	2 TTS-2 and 1 TTS-1	2 TTS-2	1 TTS-3	1 TTS-2	None

TTS-1, 0.1 mg/24 hours; TTS-2, 0.2 mg/24 hours; TTS-3, 0.3 mg/24 hours.

days, especially for those taking longer half-life opioids (e.g., methadone), one can switch to the clonidine patch and maintain for weeks, if indicated.

Before prescribing the clonidine transdermal patch, be certain the patient's diastolic blood pressure is >70 mm Hg and that he or she has no other symptoms of hypotension. As an example, continue prescribing the oral dose for one day while proceeding as follows (this should be used as a template, with individualization as dictated by blood pressure and severity of symptoms; Table 4.6): For the shorter acting opioids, the withdrawal symptoms usually start in 6–24 hours after the last dose, peak in 1–3 days, and subside within 7 days (the patient should try to not use the patch with these drugs). For the longer acting opioids, withdrawal begins within 1–3 days, peaks within 3–6 days, and subsides within 2 or more weeks (the patch will yield much more consistent results and be easier to manage in this scenario). This information is also useful for your patients. Knowing the timeline can help reassure them during this often uncomfortable process.

During this protocol, one must also consider the use of adjunctive medications, as the protocol might not be adequate to cover all symptoms. The following can be used:

- Nonsteroidal antiinflammatory drugs for pain
- Imodium for diarrhea
- Liquid antacid every 2 hours as needed for indigestion
- Regular diet as tolerated

For those patients about whom you feel uncomfortable detoxing, refer for inpatient detoxification (always a reasonable option). In this regard, for example, you might feel uncomfortable with the amount of drug being abused or you might have significant concerns relating to the veracity of the history without having the ability to corroborate the information given. Also, secondary to insurance restrictions and/or to bed capacity limits, your patient may be discharged before he or she is finished with the actual detox necessary (especially with the longer half-life opioids) and might present to your office with continuing symptoms. This scenario places your patient at a much higher risk for relapse. In this case, you will have to titrate clonidine using the above protocol (depending on the severity of symptoms, you might begin at the lowest comfortable dose possible, i.e., consider starting at a week 2 schedule).

Another protocol that can be a good alternative utilizes the GABA agonist baclofen. This medication is not often used, but it has been shown not only to be as effective as clonidine but also to have fewer problematic side effects, that is, a low incidence of hypotension (11). Therefore, if your patient is unable to tolerate clonidine, you can follow this protocol for baclofen:

- Day 1: 10 mg orally twice a day (bid)
- Day 2: 10 mg orally tid
- Day 3: 10 mg orally qid
- Days 4–7: 10 mg orally qid as needed

At this point, a word about methadone is important. This is a long half-life Schedule II medication (approximately 20 hours) that is highly regulated for methadone maintenance treatment and use in detoxification. However, its use in pain management is both reasonable (when used appropriately) and recently popular. A methadone maintenance treatment program can be a highly successful means by which to treat patients whose disease has become terminal (i.e., treatment failures with morbidity, death, and/or injury to self or others is likely). Detox for a patient on methadone maintenance treatment is usually best handled through the treatment program or via an inpatient process.

When your patient has been treated with methadone for chronic pain, a slow reduction is important for both comfort and compliance purposes. Decreasing 1–3 mg per week (or longer) is preferable, as an individual on long-term methadone treatment is more prone to have a difficult detox. In fact, the lower the dose achieved (especially below 30 mg), one author (R.P.) has found that an increasingly slow weaning process is required. If for some reason this process, even if very slow, is too uncomfortable for your patient, you can prescribe clonidine 0.1 mg by mouth up to three times per day as needed for withdrawal symptoms after you perform an in-office test dose of 0.1 mg and a blood pressure check after 1 hour. Utilization of buprenorphine for this purpose is discussed later in this chapter.

Polysubstance Dependence

Many, if not the majority, of addicts and alcoholics use multiple substances. As previously stated, obtaining a valid history is important. You cannot assume the history your patient gives is going to be reliable, and, when possible, obtaining corroborating information from the patient's close friend or relative can be very beneficial. Of course, a UDS is critical. Some basic guidelines regarding the management of polysubstance dependence are recommended:

- A patient using alcohol and benzodiazepines, if the benzodiazepine use is not high dosage, can be detoxed via the benzodiazepine protocol alone.
- For patients using alcohol and opiods, we recommend utilizing the alcohol protocol first and warning your patients to stop the opioids they are taking and prescribe Darvon 65 mg every 4 hours. After the alcohol detox is complete, discontinue the Darvon and start the clonidine protocol. To avoid potential hepatic complications, do not give Darvocet secondary to the acetaminophen. We cannot recommend strongly enough that you give only one day's worth of Darvon at a time during the procedure.

- A patient using both opioids and benzodiazepines should be referred to inpatient detox.
- Of course, use your own level of comfort to determine if the patient, in any of the above scenarios, should be referred to inpatient detox. However, again realize that the inpatient detox might not be complete and you will then have to restart a protocol after the patient is discharged back to your care from that setting.

Cocaine, Amphetamines, Marijuana, Hallucinogens, and Inhalants

No specific detox exists for cocaine, amphetamines, marijuana, hallucinogens, and inhalants. If your patient has been using stimulants (cocaine or amphetamines) and/or marijuana with alcohol, benzodiazepines, or opioids and has agreed to stop the use of all substances, you can implement the specific protocols as described previously without regard to the prior stimulant and/or marijuana use.

Intoxication episodes and potential medical complications of these substances might have to be referred to the emergency room. Much reassurance will be necessary when assessing an individual under the influence of these substances. The details regarding the management of the complications secondary to intoxication from these substances is beyond the scope of this book, and we refer you to one of the addiction medicine text books (8).

Pharmacologic Agents Used to Assist in Maintaining Abstinence

Assuming your patient has been successfully detoxed and has committed to abstinence, in addition to services offered by community-based recovery groups such as the 12 Step programs (discussed in Chapter 2), there are a few pharmacologic agents that can be of assistance to your patient. At the time of this printing, the only research-based recommended agents are for alcohol and opioids (Table 4.7).

Buprenorphine

We briefly discuss this relatively new agent approved for the use of opioid maintenance and/or detox. Buprenorphine has been available in the form of Buprenex for the treatment of pain. However, it was not until the Federal Drug Treatment Act of 2000 (12) was passed that two other forms of the drug, Suboxone and Subutex, became available. These medications are approved for use in maintenance and/or detoxification for the opioid addict. The concept basic to their approval was to provide greater access to maintenance through primary care physicians than was available through methadone maintenance clinics. However, in order to prescribe these Schedule III drugs, you must qualify for and obtain a U.S. Drug Enforcement Administration (DEA) waiver (allowing you to be assigned a Unique Identification Number as a qualified and prescribing physician; see www.samhsa.gov for complete information on the criteria you must meet in order to obtain the waiver). We limit our discussion of these medications to some basic facts and recommendations, as most non-ASAM (American Society of Addiction Medicine or subspecialty board certification from the American Osteopathic Association) certified primary care physicians will have to obtain at least 8 hours of training.

Also of note is the question regarding the use of Subutex and Suboxone for the treatment of pain. This would be an off-label use and, according to the DEA (http://asam.org/DEAPAINMANAGEMENT.html), would not be subject to the rules under DATA2000 (12). Therefore, any licensed physician with a DEA registration allowing him or her to prescribe Schedule III drugs would be allowed to prescribe these medications for the treatment of pain but, unless a waiver is obtained, would not be allowed to prescribe them for the treatment of opioid addiction. Our discussion of the use of these medications for the treatment of pain is also limited to basic facts and recommendations.

Recall that buprenorphine is a partial mu agonist that binds tightly to the receptor with a terminal half-life of approximately 32 hours. Because buprenorphine is a partial agonist with most of its activity on the mu receptor, there are inherent limits to the degree of euphoria that it can give, and it tends to plateau well below that of a full agonist. Also, secondary to its tight receptor binding, buprenorphine "kicks off" most other mu agonists from the receptor sites. Therefore, there are apparent inherent advantages to buprenorphine regarding abuse potential because of the limits of potential euphoria and it causing withdrawal symptoms in one addicted to a full agonist.

Two forms of buprenorphine are now approved for use by the opioid-addicted individual; both types are given sublingually. Suboxone is a 4 : 1 combination of buprenorphine and naloxone and Subutex (buprenorphine without naloxone). When given sublingually, the naloxone is destroyed in the stomach and does not interfere with the pharmacodynamics of the buprenorphine. However, if one attempts to inject Suboxone, the naloxone maintains its antagonist properties and precipitates withdrawal. Therefore, this combination further limits its abuse potential.

To date, buprenorphine appears at least as safe as methadone in pregnancy (13). However, secondary to the risks inherent to the fetus if the mother should experience withdrawal symptoms, it is preferable to utilize Subutex during pregnancy.

On two occasions one of the authors (R.P.) would recommend using buprenorphine for detox purposes: (1) detox from a long half-life full mu agonist, such as methadone; and (2) detox from buprenorphine. Detoxing from methadone via buprenorphine can be difficult, as one should either wait until

Table 4.7. Pharmacologic agents used to maintain abstinence (read entire prescribing information prior to using).

Drug	Indications	Mechanism of action	Effect	Contraindications	Drug interactions
Antabuse (disulfiram)	Treatment of refractory alcohol dependence	Alcohol–alcohol dehydrogenase $\rightarrow$ acetaldehyde –aldehyde dehydrogenase $\rightarrow$ $CO_2 + H_2O$	Flushing (violent), dyspnea, headache, palpitations, tachycardia, nausea/vomiting after ingestion of even small amounts of alcohol	Coronary heart disease, congestive heart failure, hypertension and history of cerebrovascular accident; *do not use in pregnancy*	Increases blood level of warfarin, phenytoin, benzodiazepines; causes change in mood or confusion with metronidazole, isoniazid, and paraldehyde; do not use with alcohol-containing substances
Campral (acamprosate)	Maintenance of abstinence from alcohol in patients with alcohol dependence	Structure similar to gamma-aminobutyric acid. Might be an N-methyl-D-aspartate receptor antagonist. Might stabilize imbalance of neurotransmitters as seen during alcohol dependence	—	Hypersensitivity, severe renal impairment (creatinine clearance ≤30 mL/min), pregnancy and nursing females	None known except weight change with antidepressants
Naltrexone	As per effect	Blocks euphorigenic effect of opioids; causes withdrawal symptoms in those dependent on opioids; reduces desire to drink alcohol in those who have stopped drinking	—	Hypersensitivity, opiate use of any kind, hepatic failure, and pregnancy	Opioids of any type. Use with caution in combination with acetaminophen and disulfiram, Mellaril, and oral hypoglycemics

Table 4.7. *Continued.*

Drug	Precautions and warnings	Laboratory tests	Dosages	Length of treatment	Cost
Antabuse (disulfiram)	Optic neuritis, peripheral neuritis, polyneuritis, peripheral neuropathy, hepatitis and hepatic failure have been reported	Baseline chemistry, complete blood count, and liver function tests; then follow up in 10–14 days, then periodically	Wait at least 24 hours after last alcohol use. Up to 50 mg each day for 1–2 weeks and then average maintenance dose is 250 mg per day. Maintenance will last months to years. The longer the treatment continues, the greater the sensitivity. No alcohol for 14 days after last dose of disulfiram	Undetermined	Approximately $40 for 250 mg (30 tablets)
Campral (acamprosate)	See contraindications	Renal function	Initiate as soon as possible after alcohol withdrawal, when the patient has achieved abstinence; should be maintained even if patient relapses: 333 mg, 2 tablets (i.e., 666 mg) three times per day with or without meals. If mild renal impairment is present, 333 mg three times per day. If severe renal impairment is present, *none*	At least 1 year	$115.49 for 333 mg tablets (180 tablets)
Naltrexone	See contraindications	Liver function tests pretreatment and periodically thereafter	Wait 7–10 days after stopping opioids; longer for methadone and levo-alpha-acetyl-methadol (levo-alpha-acetyl-methadol is rarely used, if at all, secondary to QTc prolongation and need to monitor electrocardiogram; therefore, it is not discussed in this book). Narcotic addiction: First dose, 25 mg, followed by 25 mg 1 hour later; after that, 350 mg per week, i.e., 50 mg per day for 7 days or 100 mg–100 mg–100 mg every M–W–F the first week; then 100–100–150 mg thereafter.* Alcoholism: First dose, 25 mg; then 50 mg per day	Evaluate every 3 months	Approximately $100 for 50 mg (30 tablets)

* For opioid addiction, naltrexone has been most successful for highly motivated addicts. Naltrexone is more successful for alcohol dependence in the general population. It is soon to be approved for alcohol dependence in an every-30-day depot form.
Very recently, an IM form of naltrexone (Vivitrol) was approved for use in those who are alcohol dependent. It is given one time IM (380 mg) every four weeks. Though not approved at this time, it is also promising for use in those who are opiod dependent. Precautions, lab tests, and length of treatment are similar to the above. We recommend reading the entire prescribing information and do not forget the 25 mg p.o. test dose before the first injection.

the patient is down to 30 mg of methadone before starting the detox protocol or, if the dose is higher, wait until the patient exhibits withdrawal symptoms before starting the detox.

Also, prior to using buprenorphine, patients need to be educated regarding indications, contraindications, and sublingual administration. In addition, observation during the first dose to ensure appropriate administration and effectiveness (or determine need for titration) is also important. Therefore, you should write a prescription for a very limited supply, send the patient to the pharmacy after you have obtained the patient's permission for you to talk with the pharmacist (Table 4.8 provides a sample consent form), and have the patient return and take the medication under your or your nurse's observation.

Two protocols can be used. The 5- to 8-day protocol is presented in Table 4.9, and the 20- to 36-day protocol is presented in Table 4.10 (14). Reduction rates should be individualized and can be slowed or temporarily maintained.

Table 4.8. Sample consent form.

1. Name of patient _____
2. Authorize: Dr. _____
3. To disclose [kind and amount of information to be disclosed]: Any information needed to confirm the validity of my prescription and for submission for payment for the prescription
4. To [name or title of the individual or organization to which disclosure is to be made]: The dispensing pharmacy to which I present my prescription or to which my prescription is called/sent/faxed, as well as to third parry payers
5. For [purpose of the disclosure]: Assuring the pharmacy of the validity of the prescription so that it can be legally dispensed and paid for
6. Date [on which this consent is signed]:
7. Signature of patient
8. Signature of parent or guardian [where required]
9. Signature of individual authorized to sign in lieu of the patient [where required]
10. This consent is subject to revocation at any time except to the extent that the program which is to make the disclosure has already taken action in reliance on it. If not previously revoked, this consent will terminate on [specific date, event, or condition]:

Termination of treatment.
(c) Expired, deficient, or false consent. A disclosure may not be made on the basis of a consent which: (1) has expired; (2) on its face substantially fails to conform to any of the requirements set forth in paragraph (a) of Federal law 42CFR; (3) is known to have been revoked; or (4) is known or through a reasonable effort could be known by the individual holding the records to be materially false. (Approved by the Office of Management and Budget under control number 0930-0099.)

Source: http://www.buprenorphine.samhsa.gov/bwns/Bup%20Guidelines.pdf.

Table 4.9. The 5- to 8-day protocol for buprenorphine detox.

Day	8-Day doses (mg)	5-Day doses (mg)
1	4–8	6
2	4–12	8
3	4–16	10
4	2–12	8
5	0–8	4
6	0–4	
7	0–2	
8	0 g	

Source: Adapted from Lintzeris N, Clark NC, Muhleisen P, et al. The National Clinical Guidelines and Procedures for the Use of Buprenorphine in the Treatment of Heroin Dependence. Canberra: National Drug Strategy, Commonwealth of Australia; 2001. By permission of the Australian Government, Department of Health and Ageing.

The more gradual the reduction rate, the better the outcome. There will be some mild withdrawal symptoms during the process. Education, reassurance, and continual reassessment should be utilized.

Discussion of induction of buprenorphine for maintenance is beyond the scope of this book. However, we strongly suggest that the reader become qualified to use this medication, as it is a very good alternative to methadone maintenance, with the understanding that treatment, other professional support as needed, and a recovery program are included in the treatment plan.

Table 4.10. The 20- to 36-day protocol for buprenorphine detox.

Day	36-Day doses (mg)	20-Day doses (mg)
1–4	16	16
5–8	14	8
9–12	12	4
13–16	10	2
17–20	8	0
21–24	6	
25–28	4	
29–32	2	
33–36	0	

Source: Adapted from Lintzeris N, Clark NC, Muhleisen P, et al. The National Clinical Guidelines and Procedures for the Use of Buprenorphine in the Treatment of Heroin Dependence. Canberra: National Drug Strategy, Commonwealth of Australia; 2001. By permission of the Australian Government, Department of Health and Ageing.

Pain Management and the Addicted Patient

Addicts and alcoholics are human and can experience acute and chronic pain. Although an in-depth discussion regarding this topic is beyond the scope of this book, some basic concepts are included. In addition to our personal recommendations, we also include many of Purdue Pharma L.P.'s for addressing addiction in the medical setting:

- *Your addicted patients should not have to suffer from pain* any more than your nonaddicted patients. However, recovery is an absolute necessity.
- *The same workup should be utilized* irrespective of your concerns regarding potential abuse of your treatment medications.
- When possible, if chronic opioid therapy is indicated (after all other avenues of treatment have been adequately tried), *a pain management consultation should be obtained.* This recommendation is not intended to preclude the primary care physician from treating chronic pain but to further document the need for this type of treatment for the recovering addict/alcoholic.
- *Methadone and buprenorphine are excellent choices to consider.* However, while both can be used for this purpose without a special license or waiver, the dosing is different from that used for maintenance. Methadone should be prescribed tid and buprenorphine bid for better pain control. Even though they are both long-acting medications, they yield better outcomes when one works with the peaks in the blood level. Also, these medications, for reasons already described, can help your patients maintain abstinence from other opioids.
- *DO NOT prescribe addictive forms of anxiolytics or sedative hypnotics.* Buspar (buspirone) for anxiety is not addictive, nor is Rozerem (ramelteon) for sleep. In addition, adjuvants should be utilized, including antidepressants (which can also be a good treatment for any anxiety disorder) when indicated.
- *Random and routine UDSs should be part of your agreement* with the patients.
- Encourage your patients to *strengthen their recovery program* by going to more 12 Step meetings, talking to their sponsors, and going to their places of worship and asking for more spiritual support. These actions can yield great benefit.
- Emphasize to your patients that *use of relaxation, meditation, acupuncture, massage and other ancillary measures* can help minimize their dosing requirements.
- *Remember, pseudoaddicts behave like addicts secondary to subtherapeutic treatment, but their drug-seeking behavior disappears when adequate pain relief is obtained.* A true addict reveals ongoing addictive behavior regardless of physician attempts to adequately treat the pain.
- *Protect your prescriptions* (maintain tight control of pads, never sign an incomplete or blank prescription, use tamper-resistant pads, *write quantity and strength in both numbers and letters*, do not imprint your license

or DEA number on the pad—write it in each time). Limit the amount of medication prescribed, and give no refills.

- *Be wary of certain red flags* (e.g., patients who are "traveling through town"; who start telling you about their lost prescription, i.e., "Doc, you won't believe this. . . ."; who repeatedly "lose" their prescriptions or who run out of medication before the refill date; who want their appointment at end of the day; who arrive after hours; who are demanding; who are not interested in a physical examination, physical therapy, or non-narcotic alternatives; who are reluctant to obtain old records; who have no health insurance and cannot recall the name of their previous physician; who recite either "textbook" symptoms or report a vague history; and who request specific drugs, such as Percocet, Lortab, Xanax, and OxyContin, by name "because I tried all of the others and they don't work.")

- *Stick to your principles.* Obtain a complete history and physical examination appropriate to the patient's complaint; document the results of the examination and the questions you asked; request photo identification and social security number; photocopy documents and put copies in the patient's chart; and call previous practitioners, pharmacists, hospitals, and get these phone numbers from a directory—*not* from the patient. Most importantly, *do not ever do anything that you feel uncomfortable doing.* In other words, do not let the patient push, bully, or manipulate you into writing a prescription that you are not comfortable with and that you cannot justify. Document why you did not write the prescription, and document your objective observations—leave out all subjective comments—of the patient's behavior.

- *Have a narcotics/benzodiazepine contract* and stick to it (see Appendix 2 for a sample contract).

- *Document, document, document!*

As discussed throughout this book, your addicted patients are experiencing a great deal of anxiety and pain—even if the distress is not of the exact nature they are describing to you in order to get their drugs. The distress that addicted patients feel results from their illness and from all of the chaotic thinking and behaving that accompany this illness. You can best help these patients by not becoming their "enabler" or "drug dealer"—even though it is often difficult to say "No." There is a saying, "A river without banks is just a puddle." The boundaries, or banks, you set with your addicted patients today will eventually assist them in "flowing" toward recovery instead of continuing to "drown" in the stagnant puddle of their disease. Sometimes the best and most compassionate thing we can do is to say "No," even though, at the time, it may be the most difficult word to utter to our patient in obvious distress.

Protracted Withdrawal

Protracted withdrawal is a phenomenon noted with many of the drugs we have discussed. The other name for this condition is *post-acute withdrawal syndrome.* The meaning of this term is clear: the withdrawal symptoms that continue for a period of time after completion of acute withdrawal. The DSM-IV-TR does not recognize this syndrome, although many professionals and much research in the addiction field recognize its existence and also its impact on relapse potential. We also see this phenomenon on a regular basis and see its correlation with relapse potential.

For a period of months (with alcohol) to years (potentially up to 2 years with benzodiazepines, opiates, cocaine, and maybe other substances), an addict/alcoholic can experience withdrawal symptoms. The symptoms are various but are often described by our patients as significant dysphoria/anxiety/discontent that feels, at times, out of control. The symptoms, early in recovery, are more severe and tend to diminish in intensity and frequency over time. These symptoms are usually self-limited if the patient does not use drugs again, and the physician does not prescribe an addictive medication (i.e., a benzodiazepine). The best recommendations are as follows: educate patients about the nature and extent of these symptoms; reassure them that the symptoms will dissipate; encourage them to do relaxation/breathing exercises and to increase recovery-related support activities; and, if allowed, include their closest support person (spouse, parent, etc.) in discussions.

Another recommendation we have specifically targets cocaine. One of the more disconcerting symptoms of cocaine withdrawal is a depression that can look like either dysthymic disorder or major depressive disorder. This level of depression can last up to 2 years when secondary to protracted withdrawal from cocaine. The symptoms can lead your patient back to drug use in search of relief. One of us (R.P.) highly recommends that, when your patient exhibits these symptoms, an antidepressant of your choosing should be prescribed and titrated as you would in the treatment of a primary depressive disorder. This author would also recommend the maintenance of a therapeutic dose of the antidepressant for a period of up to 2 years before considering discontinuation. This recommendation, along with the above recommendations, might mean the difference between relapse and recovery.

Last, but certainly not least, many individuals for a period of time after cessation of drug/alcohol use have difficulty with sleep, whether it is initial, middle, or terminal insomnia. Do not fall into the trap of prescribing anything that has an abuse potential; in the long run, the risks far outweigh the benefits.

Some nonpharmaceutical approaches should be attempted first. Educate and reassure your patient that for most people this is a temporary problem and that returning to drug use for relief is not a reasonable option. Learning relaxation techniques, as described in Chapter 5, is important, as is working with their sponsors to gain specific recovery-oriented coping skills. In addition, practicing sleep hygiene principles can be helpful. The following are a few sleep hygiene strategies that we often recommend to our patients:

- Turn the clock around so you cannot see what time it is.
- If you cannot sleep, get out of bed and read in a chair. When you get sleepy, go back to bed. If you still cannot fall asleep, get out of bed again. Continue to do this until you fall asleep (the bed should be used *only* for sleeping and sex).

- Do not exercise several hours before bed (but do start a regular program of exercise—this can aid in reducing insomnia).
- Do not ingest caffeine (colas, chocolate, aspirin, etc.) for several hours before bedtime. In fact, it is recommended that you reduce your overall intake of caffeine throughout the day, too.
- Do not nap during the day—no matter how sleepy you are.
- If medically indicated, have a *small* bowl of low-sugar cereal with milk an hour before bedtime. Be careful not to eat too much cereal or other foods before bed, as a very full stomach may cause you to become uncomfortable and hence increase your difficulty in falling asleep.
- Practice diaphragmatic breathing and relaxation techniques (described in Chapter 5) when you lie down for bed.
- Take a *warm* shower or bath an hour or so before bedtime (make sure the water is not too hot or too cold—extremes in temperature may stimulate you and cause you to become less sleepy).
- Go to bed and awaken at the same time 7 days a week.

It is important to realize that once patients stop taking drugs, until a good recovery program is established, and maybe even beyond this level of recovery, certain of their excessive behaviors and needs do not necessarily disappear. As this relates to sleep, your patient might consume excessive amounts of caffeine, in the form of coffee or colas, and late night activities might continue despite not going to parties or bars. Therefore, obtaining a history concerning leisure-time activities, exercise, and caffeine/sugar intake is very important.

If the above options do not help your patient to achieve the desired goal, pharmacologic intervention might *also* be necessary. One of us (R.P.) has found that trazodone 25–200 mg at bedtime can be beneficial. This medication has little abuse potential, and the side effect profile at this dose range is usually not problematic (although one must educate about the law risk of priapism). Depending on the age and health of the individual, the author often initially prescribes 50 mg and reassesses after several nights. Most patients do not require much more than 100–150 mg for appropriate sleep induction and maintenance without a "hangover." As you might already know, antidepressant doses for this medication range from 400 to 600 mg.

A relatively new medication that shows considerable promise is Rozerem (ramelteon). This drug binds selectively to the melatonin MT1 and MT2 receptors. It is not addictive, and there is only one dose of 8 mg to be given without titration. This medication has a relatively safe side effect profile, and tolerance is not a problem. However, it can take one or more weeks to determine its effectiveness.

Avoid antihistaminic agents. Addicts and alcoholics, in our experience, have a tendency to like the effect. In fact, we have seen many a relapse due to these agents. Also, be certain to educate your patient to avoid any alcohol-containing medication (remember, liquid Nyquil is 50 proof!).

If the sleep problem continues for more than a few months (or sooner if other symptoms emerge), further assessment to rule out another etiology is indicated. Be especially sensitive to the high comorbidity rate of addiction and depression or other mood disorders. Sleep is often a significant complaint with these disorders, and further questioning might reveal the presence of neuroveg-etative or other symptoms that would require more specific treatment.

Nicotine Dependence

We have left our discussion of nicotine dependence for last not because of order of importance but, from a societal and a pharmacologic perspective, nicotine is somewhat unique. This drug is legal, but, unlike alcohol, it is usually smoked. As previously discussed, this type of administration is the most addictive. Added to inhalation, the typical smoking behavior (repetitive hand to mouth, cigarette to lips, and inhalation) and immediate gratification obtained are reinforcing properties that heighten the addictive nature of this drug and make cessation very difficult.

According to the National Institute of Drug Abuse's *Infofacts*, nicotine is one of the most heavily used addictive drugs in the United States (15). In 2004, 29.2% of the U.S. population aged 12 years and older—70.3 million people—used tobacco at least once in the month prior to being interviewed. This figure includes 3.6 million young people aged 12 to 17 years. Young adults aged 18 to 25 years reported the highest rate of current use of any tobacco products (44.6%) in 2004. In addition, according to the 2003 National Survey on Drug Abuse, an estimated 35.7 million Americans were classified as nicotine dependent: 15% aged 12 years or older; 4.75% aged 12 to 17 years; 18.9% aged 18 to 25 years; and 15.8% aged 26 years and older. Unfortunately, in our experience, it is not uncommon to find the drug-addicted patient also to be addicted to nicotine.

As a primary cause of medical complications smoking is significant, and, according to the Centers for Disease Control and Prevention (CDC), tobacco use remains the leading preventable cause of death in the United States, causing approximately 440,000 premature deaths each year and resulting in an annual cost of more than $75 billion in direct medical costs attributable to smoking (16). In addition, also according to the CDC, nonsmokers exposed to secondhand smoke at home or at work have a 25% to 30% increased risk of developing heart disease and a 20% to 30% increased risk of developing lung cancer. Children exposed to secondhand smoke are at an increased risk for sudden infant death syndrome, acute respiratory infections, ear problems, and more severe asthma.

The most important part of the assessment of your patients' nicotine use is to ask direct questions. A history and physical examination should not be considered complete without having asked about a smoking or other tobacco product history. Aside from the requisite other physical and laboratory studies indicated at the time of your patient's visit, an important consideration must be given to the children in the home of a smoker, especially if the family members are suffering the sequelae of secondhand smoke. This is such an important point that if your patient states that he or she has quit, random urine cotinine (the metabolite of nicotine) levels should be obtained as support for your patient's abstinence and confirmation.

The following items can be beneficial in guiding your patient through the process of quitting:

- Use the motivational enhancement examples described in Chapter 5 to assist your patient in preparing to quit. Part of this process should include your patient being clear about the reasons to quit and being educated as to why quitting is so hard.

- Have or help the patient devise a step-by-step plan to quit.
- Provide complete information regarding the options for medication.
- Encourage your patient to do the following:
  - Set a quit day.
  - Rally support by informing as many family and friends as possible.
  - Develop a plan to manage cravings once smoking is quit.
  - Begin practicing relaxation, breathing, and other stress management techniques prior to and in preparation for the quit day and beyond.
- The following intervention may be helpful for your patient who truly wants to stop smoking but who is a habitual relapser. (It is strongly recommended that you first have a very positive, supportive relationship with the patient before initiating this behavioral contract.) Have your patient identify the organization that he or she feels most *negatively* toward (i.e., the group or organization whose principles and/or actions are the most distasteful to the patient). Then have the patient sign a contract agreeing that if he or she smokes even one cigarette, he or she will send that organization $10. Many of one of the author's (H.P.'s) patients have been able to resist their strong impulse to light up a cigarette when they have agreed to such a contract. In other words, instead of "reacting" (smoking), they "think it through" and "act" (decide not to smoke) because of this aversive consequence.

As a primary care physician, you will possibly be your patient's best source of information and support. If your patient has Internet access, there are many helpful Web sites available, for example, www.smokefree.gov. If Internet access is not an option, you may be the only source of information. Of course, the pharmaceutical companies who supply the medications used for nicotine dependence can also be an excellent source of information.

In this regard, there are multiple medications available to assist your patients in quitting smoking:

- Those that require a prescription
  - Nicotrol Nasal Spray
  - Nicotrol Inhaler
  - Zyban (bupropion SR)
- Those that do not require a prescription
  - Nicotine gum, 2 mg for a habit of fewer than 25 cigarettes/day
  - Nicotine gum, 4 mg for a habit of greater than 25 cigarettes/day
  - Commit lozenge, 2 and 4 mg
  - Patches: Nicoderm CQ, 7, 14, and 21 mg/24 hours; Nicotrol, 5, 10, and 15 mg/24 hours

It is strongly recommended for each of the above medications that you follow the manufacturer's instructions. In addition, some areas have Smokers Anonymous and/or Nicotine Anonymous meetings, which can be great non-pharmacologic supports for your patients who want to stop smoking.

Finally, most individuals do not quit after the first attempt. Being nonjudgmental and supportive is important. Review the weaknesses in your patient's plan for stopping and the problems encountered in the implementation of the plan. Encourage your patient to readjust the plan and start the steps again while realizing that each "relapse" can be a vital learning tool to achieving permanent abstinence from tobacco. For more information on nicotine dependence, refer to the excellent articles cited here (17,18).

Special Populations: Patients with Comorbid Psychiatric Disorders, Pregnant Women, Adolescents, and Older Adults

This text focuses mainly on adults with substance use disorders. Many of the principles outlined in this book, and the nonpharmacologic interventions described in Chapter 5, can be applied to your work with special populations, such as patients with a substance use disorder who have another psychiatric disorder (i.e., are "dually diagnosed"), pregnant women, adolescents, and elderly adults. In particular, many of your patients with a substance use disorder will also present with symptoms consistent with a diagnosis of another psychiatric disorder. Results from several National Institute of Drug Abuse studies suggest that the most common disorders that co-occur with substance use disorder are personality, anxiety, and mood disorders (19).

It will be important for you to differentiate between the direct effects of the substance (under the influence), acute withdrawal, or post-acute withdrawal symptoms and what is a comorbid psychiatric disorder. A general rule of thumb used by many addiction professionals is to wait as long as possible after the patient ceases substance use before diagnosing a comorbid psychiatric disorder (i.e., it may take a long time for the abnormal neurophysiologic responses caused by years of drug use to normalize—see earlier discussion of post-acute withdrawal syndrome in this chapter). However, this should not stop you from prescribing a selective serotonin reuptake inhibitor antidepressant if symptoms of depression and/or anxiety are moderate to severe. One should consider benzodiazepines and other sedative hypnotic medications to be contraindicated for the addicted population without extensive consultation with either an addictionist or addiction psychiatrist.

Differentiating between a substance use disorder and another psychiatric disorder can be difficult. Three general rules of thumb regarding differential diagnosis are presented:

- Take a good substance use history to assess when your patient's mood or other symptoms began. A comorbid disorder may be present if the symptoms began prior to the substance use.
- If the patient has a positive family history of psychiatric illness, your patient may be more likely to have a comorbid diagnosis.

- Assess whether or not your patient has had a significant "drug-free" period (of at least several months to rule out distress or other symptoms secondary to withdrawal) since he or she started using substances. If so, assess whether the same or similar psychiatric symptoms were present during that period of time. If the symptoms were present, your patient may have a co-occurring disorder. However, the symptoms may also be due to post-acute withdrawal syndrome, which can last up to 6 months and even up to 2 years in some cases. As previously mentioned, in our experience, post-acute withdrawal symptoms often improve to some degree over time and are often more intermittent. In addition, post-acute withdrawal symptoms do not necessarily follow the natural course as one would expect with a primary psychiatric disorder.

Although a discussion of the recognition and management of patients with comorbid psychiatric disorders, as well as other special populations, is beyond the scope of this book, Table 4.11 presents resources for more information. Most of the resources are from the National Library of Medicine and are available online free of charge.

Table 4.11. Resources for more information on substance abuse by patients with comorbid psychiatric disorders and/or in other special populations.

- TIP 42: Substance Abuse Treatment for Persons with Co-Occurring Disorders. Available at: http://www.ncbi.nlm.nih.gov/books/bv.fcgi?rid=hstat5.chapter.74073
- Pagano J, Graham NA, Frost-Pineda K, Gold MS. The physician's role in recognition and treatment of alcohol dependence and comorbid conditions. Psychiatr Ann 2005;35(6):473–481
- TIP 26: Substance Abuse Among Older Adults. Available at: http://www.ncbi.nlm.nih.gov/books/bv.fcgi?rid=hstat5.chapter.48302
- Rigler SK. Alcoholism in the elderly. Am Fam Physician 2000;61:1710–1716.
- TIP 31: Screening and Assessing Adolescents for Substance Use Disorders. Available at: http://www.ncbi.nlm.nih.gov/books/bv.fcgi?rid=hstat5.chapter.54841
- TIP 32: Treatment of Adolescents with Substance Use Disorders. Available at: http://www.ncbi.nlm.nih.gov/books/bv.fcgi?rid=hstat5.chapter.56031
- Leadership to Keep Children Alcohol Free (for children 9–15 years old). Available at: http://www.alcoholfreechildren.org/gs/pubs/html/Prev.htm
- TIP 2: Pregnant, Substance-Using Women. Available at: http://www.ncbi.nlm.nih.gov/books/bv.fcgi?rid=hstat5.chapter.22442
- Gold MS, Byars JA, Frost-Pineda K, Pusey AE. Substance Use in Women. In Special Issues in Women's Health. Washington, DC: American College of Obstetricians and Gynecologists; 2005:105–150
- TIP 24: A Guide to Substance Abuse Services for Primary Care Clinicians. Available at: http://www.ncbi.nlm.nih.gov/books/bv.fcgi?rid=hstat5.chapter.45293
- National Institute on Alcohol Abuse and Alcoholism: professional education materials (manuals, monographs, reports) and publications for physicians, social workers, clinicians, and other health care professionals. Available at: http://www.niaaa.nih.gov/Publications/EducationTrainingMaterials/default.htm

Multicultural Issues

Primary care physicians can play an extraordinarily important role in the elimination of the health disparities that, unfortunately, run rampant in the area of substance abuse and dependence. Although your choice of pharmacologic interventions and protocols may not differ significantly among racial, ethnic, and cultural groups, it is extremely important for you to be aware of differences among minority populations when assessing and nonpharmacologically managing addicted patients. Adequately addressing this topic is beyond the scope of this book, and we refer you to several excellent resources for more information (20–23). (We give special thanks to Jeffrey Ring, PhD, for providing references and excellent suggestions for this section.)

Referral to an Addictionist or an Addiction Psychiatrist

As discussed throughout this book, addicted patients are extremely difficult to manage. Addictionists are physicians from all specialties who are certified by the American Society of Addiction Medicine. Addiction psychiatrists are board certified by the American Board of Psychiatry and Neurology in addiction psychiatry and are specially trained in treating both the substance use disorder and any co-occurring psychiatric disorders. It is our recommendation that you contact an addictionist or an addiction psychiatrist in your

Table 4.12. Sources for finding local addictionists and addiction psychiatrists.

American Society of Addiction Medicine (ASAM)
4601 N. Park Avenue
Upper Arcade #101
Chevy Chase, MD 20815
Phone: 301-656-3920
Fax: 301-656-3815
e-mail: email@asam.org
Web site: http://www.asam.org/

American Academy of Addiction Psychiatry
1010 Vermont Avenue, NW, Suite 710
Washington, DC 20005
Phone: 202-393-4484
Fax: 202-393-4419
Web site: http://www.aaap.org/home.htm

area to assist you with the management of your addicted patients. Many of these professionals have practices that also offer services such as evaluation/ consultation, individual and group psychotherapy and case management, as well as placement in drug treatment centers. Addictionists/Addiction Psychiatrists in your area can be accessed through the resources presented in Table 4.12. When treating patients with substance use disorders, it is important to know that you do not have to do it alone.

References

1. Dupont RL, Gold MS. Withdrawal and reward: implications for detoxification and relapse prevention. Psychiatr Ann 1995;25(11):663–668.
2. Adinoff B, O'Neill HK, Ballenger JC. Alcohol withdrawal and limbic kindling: a hypothesis of relapse. Am J Addict 1995;4:5–17.
3. Saitz R. Unhealthy alcohol use. N Engl J Med 2005;352:596–607.
4. Heilig M, Egli M. Pharmacological treatment of alcohol dependence: target symptoms and target mechanisms. Pharmacol Ther 2006;111:855–876.
5. Miller L, Greenblatt DJ, et al. Chronic benzodiazepine administration I: tolerance is associated with benzodiazepine receptor down regulation and decreased GABA receptor function. J Pharmacol Exp Ther 1988;246(1):170–176.
6. Miller L, Greenblatt DJ, et al. Chronic benzodiazepine administration II: discontinuation syndrome is associated with up regulation of GABA receptor complex binding and function. J Pharmacol Exp Ther 1988;246(1):177–181.
7. Miller L. Chronic benzodiazepine administration: from patient to gene. J Clin Pharmacol 1991;31:492–495.
8. Graham AW, Schultz TK, eds. Principles of Addiction Medicine, 2nd ed. Chevy Chase, MD: American Society of Addiction Medicine; 1998.
9. Gold M, Redmond DE, Kleber HD. Clonidine blocks acute opiate withdrawal symptoms. Lancet 1978;2:599–600.
10. Gold MS, Pottash AC, Sweeney DR, Kleber HD. Opiate withdrawal using clonidine. JAMA 1980;243:343–346.
11. Ahmadi-Abhari SA, Akhondzadeh S, Assadi SM, Shabestari OL, Farzanehgan ZM, Kamlipour A. Baclofen versus clonidine in the treatment of opiates withdrawal, side-effects aspect: a double-blind randomized controlled trial. J Clin Pharm Ther 2001;26:67–71.
12. Drug Addiction Treatment Act of 2000 (DATA 2000). Title XXXV, Section 3502 of the Children's Health Act of 2000. Waiver Authority for Physicians Who Dispense or Prescribe Certain Narcotic Drugs for Maintenance Treatment or Detoxification Treatment. Public Law 106–310 106th Congress, An Act. Available at: http:// buprenorphine.samhsa.gov/fulllaw.html.
13. Johnson RE, Jones HE, Fischer G. Use of buprenorphine in pregnancy: patient management and effects on the neonate. Drug Alcohol Depend 2003;70:S87–S101.

14. Johnson RE, Strain EC, Amas L. Buprenorphine: how to use it right. Drug Alcohol Depend 2003;70:559–577.
15. InfoFacts: Cigarettes and Other Tobacco Products. Bethesda, MD: National Institute on Drug Abuse. Revised July 11, 2006. Available at: http://www.drugabuse.gov/infofacts/tobacco.html.
16. The Office on Smoking and Health. Tobacco Information and Prevention Source. National Center for Chronic Disease Prevention and Health Promotion, Centers for Disease Control and Prevention. 2006. Available at: http://www.cdc.gov/tobacco/issue.htm.
17. Schroeder SA. What to do with a patient who smokes. JAMA 2005;294(4):482–487.
18. Gold MS, Edwards DW. Treating cigarette smokers in 2000. Your Patient Fitness 2000;14(4);6–11.
19. Leshner AI. Drug abuse and mental disorders: co-morbidity is reality [director's column]. NIDA Notes 1999;14(4). Available at: http://www.nida.nih.gov/NIDA_Notes/NNVol14N4/DirRepVol14N4.html.
20. Krestan J-A. Bridges to Recovery: Addiction, Family Therapy and Multicultural Treatment. New York: The Free Press; 2000.
21. Straussner SLA, ed. Ethnocultural Factors in Substance Abuse Treatment. New York: The Guilford Press; 2002.
22. Primm B, Brown L Jr, Primm A, Friedman J. Tobacco, alcohol and drugs. In Satcher D, Pamies R, eds. Multicultural Medicine and Health Disparities. New York: McGraw-Hill; 2006.
23. Cooper L. Drug Use Among Racial/Ethnic Minorities. Bethesda, MD: National Institute on Drug Abuse, provided scientific oversight, critical review, and substantive comments for this publication, revised 2003. For questions or comments on this documents, please send an e-mail to De. Leslie Cooper at: lc58q@nih.gov. Available at: www.drugabuse.gov.

5. Nonpharmacologic Office-Based Interventions: Cognitive-Behavioral Therapy and Motivational Interviewing

There are myriad nonpharmacologic interventions that are used in traditional addiction treatment, ranging from individual and group psychotherapies, to self-control and social skills training, to aversion therapies. However, despite the vast array of treatment strategies, the literature suggests that when it comes to treating substance addiction, no one modality is superior to any other (1). Rather, there are a variety of treatments, and combinations of treatments, that can be helpful for the addicted patient. Unfortunately, for the majority of primary care physicians, obstacles such as limited time and lack of training in this area make the implementation of traditional interventions unfeasible. This chapter gives the physician an overview of two well-known and well-studied brief nonpharmacologic interventions—cognitive-behavioral therapy (CBT) and motivational interviewing (MI)—that can be administered by the physician in an office-based setting.

Indeed, the treatment modality with the greatest amount of empirical support regarding effectiveness are brief interventions. In a recent study that used elements of both CBT and MI with a sample of human immunodeficiency virus–positive adults with a substance use disorder, it was demonstrated that these interventions significantly decreased substance use in this population (2). In addition, Baker et al. (3) found that a brief intervention consisting of CBT and MI increased the likelihood of abstinence from amphetamines in a group of regular amphetamine users and that this reduction in use was also accompanied by significant improvements in stage of change (discussed in the next section), benzodiazepine use, tobacco smoking, polydrug use, injection risk behavior, criminal activity level, and psychiatric distress and depression level. Bertholet et al. (4) reviewed 19 trials that included 5,639 outpatients from primary care clinics. These researchers found that brief alcohol interventions administered in the primary care setting are effective in reducing alcohol consumption.

In the 15 minutes allotted for most patient visits in primary care, the fact that brief interventions can be very effective in helping addicted patients is good news. In 1990, the Institute of Medicine concluded that brief interventions are appropriate interventions to treat substance abusers outside of the specialized drug treatment sector (e.g., for implementation by primary care physicians and psychiatrists in general practice [1]).

Elements of both CBT and MI can be used by the primary care physician to assist with the overall treatment of addicted patients. In addition, it is hoped that by gaining knowledge about these interventions, physicians will experience a greater sense of perceived control by virtue of being better equipped to deal with these very difficult patients. In Appendix 1, we use a case example to present and integrate strategies from both frameworks into a practical, patient-focused approach.

Brief Overview of Theory: Cognitive-Behavioral Therapy and Motivational Interviewing

Cognitive-Behavioral Therapy

Cognitive-behavioral therapy is one of the most widely used and studied interventions in primary care. Cognitive therapy developed from Dr. Aaron Beck's early research on depression (5–7). Beck found that, contrary to Freud's view that depression was anger turned inward, it was themes of defeat—not anger—that were evident in patients' dialogues (8). Beck proposed that "an organism needs to process information in an adaptive way in order to survive. Much of this processing is automatic and outside of awareness. Further, this process is not necessarily rational (or) logical" (8).

Albert Ellis, another contributor to cognitive therapy vis-à-vis his "rational-emotive therapy" approach, says it more simply, "We feel what we think" (9). This, then, is the essence of CBT: our thoughts are created because of our perceptions about situations (people, places, and events), and these thoughts, in turn, create feelings. From a medical psychology perspective, feelings then influence our physical sensations by activating the sympathetic nervous system and the "fight or flight" response. Our feelings, and the accompanying physical sensations, then affect the choices we make (behaviors).

This can be best illustrated by the struggle faced by most patients who are living with chronic pain. People's perceptions of a situation as threatening their available coping resources leads to distressful feelings, which leads to tightening muscles and increased blood pressure, which leads to greater perceptions of pain, which leads to short-term rewarding, long-term defeating behaviors (greater use of narcotics, avoidance behaviors that, in the long run, make pain worse, etc.), which leads to more negative thoughts, which leads to more distressful feelings, and so on. It is as if these patients are like hamsters on a wheel: the cognitive-emotional-physical-behavioral cycle continues and the patients lose hope in ever freeing themselves from this wheel of negativity and pain (Figure 5.1).

The problem is, as Beck described and as is illustrated in Figure 5.1, this processing is not always rational—even in "high-functioning," nonaddicted individuals. There are a variety of ways that individuals distort—or exhibit errors in—their thinking processes. Although there are many types of cognitive errors (see Persons [10] for a succinct review), we focus on three major cognitive distortions: dichotomous thinking, personalization, and overgeneralization.

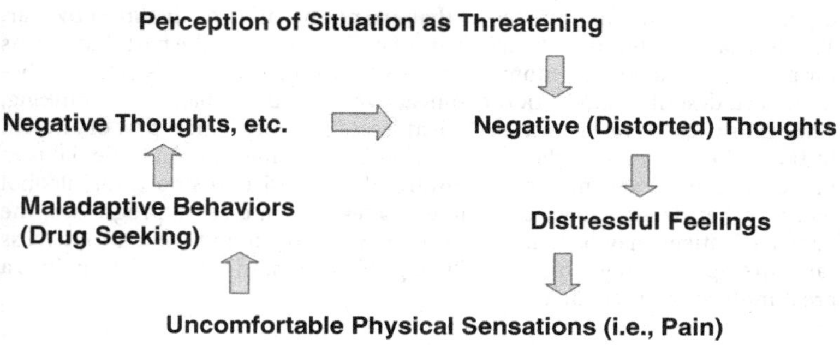

Perception of Situation as Threatening

⬇

Negative Thoughts, etc. ⟹ **Negative (Distorted) Thoughts**

⬆

Maladaptive Behaviors (Drug Seeking)

⬇

Distressful Feelings

⬆

⬇

Uncomfortable Physical Sensations (i.e., Pain)

Figure 5.1. Relationships among situations, negative thoughts, distressful feelings, physical sensations (pain), and maladaptive behaviors.

Dichotomous thinking occurs when one categorizes experiences into one of two extremes, for example, "all good" or "all bad." For example, your patient may either feel that everything is "great" or that everything is "terrible"; there are no gray areas in between these opposite poles (dichotomous thinking is also referred to as "polarization" or "black or white thinking").

Personalization is evident when patients can only think in terms of themselves and attribute external events to themselves in the absence of any causal connection. For example, after being given a mean look by a stranger in the elevator on the way to his appointment with you, your patient states, "I knew that he didn't like me, probably because I didn't look very neat this morning. I should have put on better clothes before coming to see you."

Unlike personalization, in which there are usually *no* data to support the patient's conclusion, the third major error, *overgeneralization*, occurs when conclusions are drawn beyond the substance of the data; in other words, data exist, but the conclusions drawn from them are faulty. For example, your patient has been criticized by her supervisor and she now reports that she feels like a "total failure" and that she will "never be able to please him or anyone else." In essence, she has formulated a general rule based on one or several isolated incidents that she is applying broadly to other situations (8). The subtle differences between these different types of cognitive errors are not as important as the understanding that even well-adjusted individuals frequently can, and do, have errors in their thinking that, in turn, create distressful feelings and physical states. Beck refers to cognitions that create uncomfortable feelings and somatic sensations as "negative self-talk." This negative inward dialogue can then lead to compensatory behaviors (aimed at reducing emotional/ physical discomfort), which are often maladaptive in nature.

Addicted patients, because of the fear-based nature of their illness, appear to exist in an almost constant state of chaotic, distorted thinking, or negative self-talk. Probably the most important goal that you, the primary care physician, can accomplish is to help your addicted patients become aware of the aspects of their thinking processes that are not negative or distorted by fear. This is what we refer to as the *wise* part of each individual, the part that yearns for peace of mind and freedom from the suffocating cage that is active addiction. Beck describes this antidote to negative self-talk as "balanced" thinking, while Ellis uses the term "rational" to address this more logical part of oneself. In the earlier stages of addiction, when the defense mechanism of denial is at its peak, your patient may not be aware of this desire to stop using alcohol and/or other drugs. However, in later stages, as the disease progresses, the addicted patient may become increasingly more open and willing to discuss (and attempt to change) his or her "using" behaviors. In other words, pain is a great motivator for change.

Motivational Interviewing

Like CBT, MI offers an extremely useful framework from which to view the addictive process. Motivational interviewing focuses on how to use the motivation that stems from pain to assist with behavior change from a "stage" perspective. The literature attesting to the beneficial effects of motivational interviewing with problem drinkers (11–14), heroin users (15), cocaine users (16), regular amphetamine users (3), and polydrug users (2) is enormous.

Motivational interviewing stems from a theoretical construct known as the transtheoretical stages-of-change model (17). This model emerged from an examination of 18 psychological and behavioral theories about how change occurs, including components that make up the biopsychosocial framework for understanding addiction (18). Put simply, a central premise of MI is that individuals move through stages of behavior change; that is, a behavior change does not occur overnight. Unfortunately, in most primary care settings and elsewhere, patients are ordered to immediately stop smoking, drinking, over-eating, and so forth. However, if change is a dynamic, time-intensive process, and not an immediate event, we can see why most primary care physicians feel so frustrated by their patient's noncompliance; quick results invariably never occur. So, the bad news is that our patients are unlikely to respond to our admonishments and take our recommendations to heart right away. The good news, though, is that by using MI strategies and by conceptualizing our patients' struggles from a stage perspective, we can help them move through the process more quickly. Equally important is that by using MI techniques in your practice, you will feel less pressured to "cure" your patients and your patients will feel more in control of their choices. The end result can be a much-improved, and therefore more mutually beneficial and effective, physician–patient relationship.

The five stages of change proposed by the transtheoretical model are (1) Precontemplation, (2) Contemplation, (3) Preparation (or Determination), (4) Action, and (5) Maintenance. These stages are not linear; that is, one does not enter one stage and go directly to the next. Rather, these stages can be conceptualized as a dynamic cycle through which patients move back and forth (Table 5.1) (18).

Table 5.1. The five stages of change.

Stages	Descriptors
1) Precontemplation	Person is not considering or does not want to change a particular behavior
2) Contemplation	Person is thinking about changing a behavior
3) Preparation/Determination	Person is seriously considering and planning to change a behavior and has taken steps toward change
4) Action	Person is actively doing things to change or modify behavior
5) Maintenance	Person continues to maintain behavioral change until it becomes permanent

Source: Data are from Prochaska and DiClemente [17] and Miller [18].

> There is a myth . . . in dealing with serious health-related addictive . . . problems, that more is always better. More education, more intense treatment, more confrontation will necessarily produce more change. Nowhere is this less true than with Precontemplators. More intensity will often produce fewer results with this group. So it is particularly important to use careful motivational strategies, rather than to mount high-intensity programs . . . that will not be ignored by those uninterested in changing the . . . problem behavior. . . . We cannot make Precontemplators change, but we can help motivate them to move to Contemplation. (DiClemente et al. [19])

During the *Precontemplation* stage, addicted patients will minimize or deny that they have a problem. Patients are not considering change at this point and do not perceive that they have experienced adverse consequences because of their substance use. This is the stage in which most of our "difficult patients" reside. It seems that everyone around the patients (family, friends, health care teams) know that the patients drink or use too much, but the patients are blind to this fact. Most physicians make the grave error of attempting to "force" the Precontemplative patient to stop drinking and/or using other substances: "You are killing yourself—you *have* to stop drinking *now*!" "You just need to quit—don't you see what your drug use is doing to you?" Statements such as these, as DiClemente et al. (19) suggested, may cause Precontemplators to withdraw and become more (rather than less) resistant to efforts to get them to stop using. While we cannot "cure" or change anyone, we *can* help the Precontemplator to move to the next stage of change: Contemplation.

> Contemplation is often a very paradoxical stage . . . (and) ambivalence can make contemplation a chronic (and extremely frustrating) condition. . . . Ambivalence is the archenemy of commitment and a prime reason for chronic contemplation. . . . (DiClemente et al. [19])

When patients begin to realize that their substance use may be problematic, they are in the *Contemplation* stage. As the name suggests, these patients are beginning to consider the "cons" of using a substance, but are still experiencing a great deal of ambivalence with regard to change. They may simultaneously see reasons to change and reasons not to change their substance use. During this stage, it may seem that they are straddling a fence, which, of course, is a very uncomfortable position to be in. As DiClemente et al. (19) noted, it can also be an extremely frustrating time for you, as the physician, because one minute these patients seem to truly want to change, and the next minute they are noncompliant with your recommendations and are drinking and ingesting drugs more than ever (in their mind, what better way to deal with ambivalence?).

However, from a clinical perspective, this discomfort of the patients may be viewed as a positive thing. Again, without a certain amount of pain and discomfort, they may not have the motivation they will need to initiate and eventually sustain long-term change.

> ... Help the [patient] work through the ambivalence [of the Contemplation stage], to anticipate the barriers, to decrease the desirability of the problem behavior, and to gain some increased sense of self-efficacy to cope with this specific problem.... (DiClemente et al. [19])

When addicted patients realize that the pros of stopping substance use outweigh the cons and they become willing to plan how to make this change come about, they have moved into the *Preparation* (also known as the *Determination*) stage. This is a time when commitment is strengthened. The patients will still be using alcohol and/or other drugs during this time, but typically they intend to stop using them very soon. Your patient may say things such as, "Okay, Doc, I am ready to stop drinking. I'm going to shoot for the end of this month" and "I've realized that I need to stop using. It's ruining my life. But, how do I stop?" Statements such as these indicate that patients are not only in the Preparation stage but are also poised to move toward Action.

> Strong commitment alone does not guarantee change. Unfortunately, enthusiasm does not make up for ineptness.... Commitment without appropriate coping skills and activities can create a tenuous action plan.... Anticipation of problems and pitfalls appears to be a solid problem-solving skill. (DiClemente et al. [19])

Patients in the *Action* stage have chosen a strategy for change and are beginning to pursue it. They have stopped using substances and may have entered a detox program and/or a drug treatment center. They may also have started attending Alcoholics or Narcotics Anonymous meetings and/or are making other drastic lifestyle changes (changing friends, avoiding old hangouts, etc.). These patients are actively working on modifying their behavior during this stage. Even though they are making positive movement, you must realize that they may also be feeling very vulnerable. They may also be experiencing the effects of withdrawal from their drug of choice. Some patients, however, may not feel vulnerable or uncomfortable at all—they may be very excited and upbeat during the earlier parts of this stage and may remark that they feel "on top of the world" or that they have finally "got this thing licked!" Miller (18) states that "[The Action stage] may last 3 to 6 months following termination or reduction of substance use. For some, it is a honeymoon period before they face more daunting and longstanding challenges."

Although Miller (18) views a "reduction" in use as a qualifier for placement in the Action stage, it should be noted at this point that we believe that once a patient crosses the line into active addiction, *successful use of any mind or mood-altering substance (even if the substance in question was not your patient's drug of choice) is not an option for healthy, long-term recovery*. We base this statement on our review of the literature, as well as on our own personal and professional experiences. We have found that "a drug is a drug is a drug," and switching substances or trying to control, or to cut down, on one's use is not effective in the long run. Eventually, the end result of switching or reducing one's substance use is almost always one of the following: (1) the addicted patient will return to the initial level of problematic use after efforts to cut down fail; (2) the addicted patient will return to the use of his other drug of choice after using a "substitute" drug (i.e., return to cocaine use after a brief period of using "only" alcohol); or (3) the drug that was used as a substitute becomes problematic (i.e., the patient is no longer using cocaine but his or her drinking is out of control). Indeed, for the clinician, it may be helpful to remember a phrase often spoken in 12 Step meetings: "the easiest part of stopping alcohol and other drugs is the stopping; the hardest part is staying stopped." Once patients have been in the Action stage for at least 6 months, they have moved into the *Maintenance* stage.

> Maintenance is not the absence of change, but the continuance of change. (Prochaska and DiClemente [17])

Maintenance is the stage in which the individual is working to maintain sobriety and to prevent recurrence, or relapse (20). Your patient will likely be experiencing a drastic decrease in both the physical craving and the mental obsession to use substances. However, he or she will still need to remain extremely vigilant and will need to become aware of and knowledgeable about the specific types of situations and triggers that may lead to a relapse (i.e., the patient should have a relapse prevention plan).

Although you do not want your patient to relapse into active substance use, the phenomenon of *Relapse* (or *Recurrence*) can be viewed as an important learning process, a process by which sobriety may actually be strengthened in the long run by breaking down any remaining reservations or resistance to the idea of living drug-free. Judging and/or admonishing a patient for a relapse can be detrimental for the individual's return to recovery as well as to the physician–patient relationship. Relapse is the event that triggers the individual's return to earlier stages of change and recycling through the process (18). After a period of sobriety, many addicted patients do revert to an earlier stage by returning to active substance use at least once.

Now that we have briefly discussed the bare bones in terms of the theoretical underpinnings of both CBT and MI, we now turn to the more practical aspects, or the meat, of these two approaches.

Strategies for the Primary Care Setting

Cognitive-Behavioral Interventions

Although there are a variety of interventions that stem from CBT theory, we focus on three strategies that are likely to be the most effective, practical, and easily translatable into an office-based primary care practice: (1) cognitive restructuring, (2) mindfulness (a "here and now" focus), and (3) diaphragmatic breathing and brief relaxation/imagery exercises. Each intervention should be introduced in one clinic visit because each builds upon the next. All of these strategies are integrated and demonstrated in three visits via case presentation in Appendix 1.

> If you are distressed by anything external, the pain is not due to the thing itself but to your own estimate of it; and this you have the power to revoke at any moment.
> Marcus Aurelius

Cognitive Restructuring (or, Getting the Monkey off Your Patient's Back)

The statement by Marcus Aurelius describes the essence of cognitive restructuring. As discussed earlier, CBT is based on the theory that thoughts create feelings that, in turn, influence physical sensations and behaviors. Cognitive restructuring is the practice of changing one's negative, distorted self-talk into more balanced, accurate cognitions. For example, your patient might remark, "I'll never be able to live without my Xanax—I am always anxious when I don't take it." Negative self-talk is often identified when certain absolutist words or phrases (red flags), such as *never* and *always*, are used. When thinking thoughts such as these, your patient is undoubtedly feeling very anxious and physiologically aroused and is probably wishing she had a Xanax right now (behavior). The term one of us (H.P.) uses to describe the incessant chatter of our negative, distorted thoughts is *monkey talk*. H.P. has been using this term for years with patients and residents and has found that the majority of individuals relate well to this metaphor—regardless of what age they are. When either H.P. or a resident is describing the monkey, patients will nod and smile in recognition. We all have a monkey. This is the part of us that is fear based, that worries about the future (the "what ifs": What if this bad thing happens? What if I don't pass my boards?) or about the past ("woulda, coulda, shoulda": I should have never done that, if only I could go back and do it over again, I would do things so differently.). H.P. teaches patients that the monkey is our enemy ("We have met the enemy and he is us"—Pogo [Walt Kelly, 1972]);

it is the aspect of our humanness that "sabotages" efforts to achieve happiness. Remember, if thoughts create feelings, then when we listen to our monkey and "what if" about the future, it is almost certain we will feel anxiety. Likewise, focusing on monkey talk detailing all of the mistakes, heartbreaks, bad choices, and past hurts will create feelings of depression, guilt, shame, resentment, regret, and remorse.

By teaching your patients about the relationships between thoughts, feelings, sensations, and behaviors, you can help them to increase their awareness of their monkey—or negative self-talk (only by becoming aware of something can we change it). Once aware, they are then able to restructure. One way of doing this is to ask your patient, "What can you tell yourself that would make you feel less anxious (or sad, scared, depressed, angry)?" Most patients will have a difficult time coming up with a balanced thought—the negativity of their monkey talk is too loud. H.P. encourages patients to identify the part of themselves that is "wise" and that "wants peace and joy—the part of you that just wants to be happy—the opposite of the negative, fear-based monkey part of yourself."

Most patients are able to acknowledge the existence of a "higher self" or a "wise self." They realize that this is the part of them that has gotten them through difficult times in their lives, the aspect of self that consistently has the answer that is the best for them on all levels. So, if patients have difficulty coming up with a balanced thought based on the question, "What can you tell yourself that would make you feel less—?" H.P. would ask, "Okay, then what would that wise part of you tell you right now about the situation?" Most patients are then able to come up with a thought to refute, or to work as an antidote against, their monkey's negative self-talk. Using the example above, your patient, might then be able to change her negative statement, "I'll never be able to live without my Xanax—I am always anxious when I don't take it." into a more balanced (and much less distressing) thought, such as, "I'm scared about the idea of getting off Xanax, but I know that is what I need to do and that I'll be okay—or, at least I believe my doctor thinks I'll be okay." Of course, your patient will not believe this new thought as much as she believes the previous, negative one. She should be reassured that this is normal and will take time and practice but that yes, her more balanced thought *is* the accurate one and the one that will aid her in breaking free of her addiction to Xanax.

It should also be noted that spirituality can have an extremely important role in assisting with successful restructuring of negative cognitions. Indeed, the literature attesting to the beneficial effects of spirituality in decreasing distress and in improving biopsychosocial outcomes is enormous (21–24). It is critical to also note that the term "spirituality" does not necessarily mean "religiosity." Patients may have a belief in a "God," "Higher Power," "mother nature," "spirit," and so on that may not fall into a particular religious framework per se. However, we believe, based on empirical data and on our own clinical experiences, that it is extremely important to ask your addicted patients about their spiritual beliefs—especially when you are teaching them cognitive restructuring. That is, if your patient believes in "something greater than himself" that is benevolent and caring, the restructuring process can become much easier. For example, after receiving an affirmative answer from your patient with regard to spiritual beliefs (and finding out what term he or she uses to describe this "greater being"), you might say, "If (God, Jehovah, Jesus, Higher Power, Mother Nature) could talk to you *right now* and you and I could hear (Him, Her, It), what would (He, She, It) tell you *right now* about the situation?" Patients find that this "(God, Higher Power, etc.) talk" is consistently the *opposite* of whatever their monkey is telling them—it is the same message that they would get from their wise self (for atheistic patients, teaching them about the wise self appears to work in the same manner that what might be termed as the "spiritual self" works for your patients who have these beliefs).

After teaching your patient how to change thoughts to change feelings, it is important to prescribe "homework" based on this newly acquired information. For example, you might instruct your patient in the following manner: "So, we've discussed how to change your thoughts to change your feelings. I would like to give you some homework to do before our next visit, if that's okay with you. First, I would like for you to simply become aware of the monkey—your negative self-talk. The way you do this is, anytime you are feeling 'bad' (anxious, sad, angry), try to become aware of what your thoughts are at that moment. Then, what I would like to suggest is that you make a decision to change monkey talk to (wise self, God, Higher Power) talk. Remember, you do this by asking 'What would — say to me right now about the situation?' Also remember that this is simple, but not easy; be gentle with yourself. Try doing this at first when you are not feeling really anxious, sad, or angry. We'll use this later to help when your feelings are really strong. For now, though, just work to change your thoughts when you are feeling a little (anxious, sad, angry, etc.)."

Make sure that you document (1) that you taught your patient cognitive restructuring; (2) what term your patient uses to describe the wiser, more balanced aspect of self; and (3) what you prescribed for homework. When your patient returns for follow-up, whether it is for a regular medical or for a stress management visit, you can focus on the homework you prescribed and identify successes and difficulties with your patient's ability to cognitively restructure negative, distorted "monkey talk." Asking about homework and/or elements of the previous visit tends to help keep the visit on track and brief—you have a goal in mind (assessing the patient's participation in homework with the aim of decreasing distress and, indirectly, the patient's substance use), and all other dialogue can be continuously brought back to this goal.

In summary, cognitive restructuring

- Is extremely useful in assisting addicted patients in reducing distressful feelings and the resultant uncomfortable physical state these emotions engender. It may also assist in curbing craving and behavioral "acting out" (i.e., reaching for a drink/drug).
- Focuses on changing negative, distorted "monkey talk" into more balanced "wise self" or "spiritual self" talk. In our experience, balanced thoughts usually appear to be the opposite of distorted thoughts.
- Is relatively "simple" to explain to patients but is not "easy" to put into practice. Reassure patients that it will take awhile to begin to truly believe the more balanced cognitions.

Finally, supplement cognitive restructuring by prescribing homework. By becoming aware of negative self-talk and then making the decision to change negative self-talk to "wise self talk/God talk," patients can become more adept in the art of cognitive restructuring and therefore less distressed. The art of teaching patients cognitive restructuring is further elaborated upon in Appendix 1.

Mindfulness ("Here and Now" Focus)

Have you ever wondered why little children seem so happy? Of course, they also fleetingly experience many other emotions (anger, sadness, fear), but they seem to keep returning to a base of happiness. The reason for this may be that most young children do not have a monkey yet. That is, the majority of kids under the age of 5 years or so do not dwell on the future, nor do they fret about the past. They are so plugged into the moment that their emotions may shift rapidly (Mommy! Look at the birdie! [excitement, glee] Will the birdie bite me? [fear] I want the birdie! [whining/frustration] Oh, another birdie! [excitement and happiness again]).

Mindfulness is a concept derived from Buddhism, and its central emphasis is on the importance of focusing on the here and now. H.P. teaches her primary care patients the "awareness exercise" on their second visit. It is a wonderful strategy to help disconnect from monkey talk in order to find a moment of respite from the negative chatter and replace this negative thinking with more balanced thoughts.

Prior to demonstrating this exercise and after drawing patients' attention to the concept that "happiness exists in the present," ask the patients to watch you for the next several seconds. When you are finished, ask them to tell you what they observed. Reassure them that "there are no wrong answers" and that "this is not a test." Then take a deep breath and simply describe everything you see, hear, feel, and, to a lesser extent taste or smell for the next 20 seconds or so. Express this sensory "inventory" in a succinct fashion with as little detail as possible. For example, "I am aware of the brown and white (colors of the floor, but only the colors are described). I hear talking outside. I see a pen. My hands feel warm. I am aware of greens and blues and reds (in a painting on the wall, but, again, only the colors are verbalized), I hear a hum," and so forth. Describe only objective facts that you can observe, hear, and feel—colors, textures, sounds (without hypothesizing the source of the sound, i.e., hum of the air conditioning, sound of the fax machine, etc.—just "the hum," or "a sound"). Patients usually smile and nod as they watch this demonstration. Perhaps on a deep level, as if hearing a faraway echo, we all remember and recognize—as if running into an old, beloved friend from the past—this sensory-oriented, here-and-now way of processing from our childhoods.

Most patients are able to identify that you are "being aware of everything around you, in the moment." Then ask the patient to "tell me what I was *not* doing." Very few patients are able to state that you were not judging, "thinking," or focusing on the future or the past; this usually has to be pointed out to them. Once pointed out, again, they nod in recognition. The majority of patients find this to be an extremely useful exercise to help them to "get out of (your) head (and away from the monkey) by grounding (you) in the moment." As with cognitive restructuring, this awareness exercise is further illustrated with a case presentation in Appendix 1.

Diaphragmatic Breathing

In addition to living in the moment, small children also tend to breathe "correctly," that is, very deeply from their diaphragms. As we grow older, it seems as if we not only forget how to live minute by minute but we also forget how to breathe. Actually, these two things may be related in that as we start listening to our monkey, we become stressed and therefore our breathing becomes more shallow and rapid. In demonstrating diaphragmatic breathing, ask your patients to put one hand on their chest and the other on their stomach (diaphragm). Make sure you physically demonstrate this by putting your own hands on these areas of your body too. Then ask the patient to "Take a really deep breath, and, while you are breathing in, pay attention to which hand moves more, the one on your chest, or the one on your stomach." Patients may need to do this a couple of times—especially obese patients—before they can get a sense of which hand is moving the most. After the patients make this distinction, explain to them that "when we are "stressed," the hand on our chest moves more. When we are relaxed, or not so stressed, the hand on our stomach, or diaphragm, moves more." Further inform the patients that they can actually reduce their stress level by taking in 10 deep breaths from their diaphragm three times each day. The less stressed addicted patients are, the greater are their chances at achieving long-term sobriety. In addition, because of the relationships between thoughts, feelings, sensations, and behaviors, this type of breathing can help relieve some of the chronic pain and/or other physical distress some patients also experience.

Brief Relaxation Exercise

After teaching patients diaphragmatic breathing, you can now introduce a brief relaxation exercise. It is a good idea to first (1) find out if the patient has ever engaged in relaxation before; (2) let the patient know that you will not be "hypnotizing" him or her, and (3) reassure the patient that you will turn away from him or her to "give you your space" (which is especially important for those patients who may have a history of abuse—it can be very disconcerting to have someone, even a trusted physician, looking at them when their eyes are closed). We also suggest telling your patients that this exercise is "very safe" and that if they want to stop and open their eyes at any time, they may do so. Finally, we suggest informing patients that there is "no right or wrong way to do this," that if they have difficulty with any part of the exercise—not to worry. Practice will make "close to perfect" (because "perfect" does not exist.) Right before beginning this exercise, ask the patient to "rate your level of (anxiety, stress, depression, etc.)."

The first part of the exercise focuses on relaxing each part of the body; the second part focuses on creating a comforting image. The goal of the exercise is to help your patients "disconnect" from their thinking, or monkey, and therefore to feel more relaxed and peaceful. You can begin this 5- to 8-minute exercise by saying something along these lines (pause for about 3 to 5 seconds wherever you see the "..."):

> Close your eyes and get into a comfortable position. I'll close my eyes too and turn away from you so you can have your "own space" ... remember, if you want to stop at any time, you may do so ... and if any thoughts or sounds distract you during the next few minutes, just gently re-focus your attention onto my voice....
>
> Take a very deep breath ... from your diaphragm as we discussed ... and imagine that your feet are in a wonderful, warm tub of water ... the water is the perfect temperature, neither too cool nor too warm ... just perfect. Take another deep breath and imagine that you have just lowered your legs, from your knees down, into this wonderful bath ... you feel very safe and warm.... Take another deep breath and allow the water to travel all the way up to your waist ... it's as if you've lowered your body from your waist down into this wonderful, soothing bath ... you feel the warmth against your lower back and you feel yourself becoming very relaxed. Take another deep breath ... and imagine that you have a warm, soft towel across your shoulders ... the weight of the towel is gently pushing your shoulders down toward the floor ... as you take another deep breath imagine you are slowly lying back in the tub ... the towel is cushioning your neck and head and you feel very relaxed and safe ... you breathe deeply and feel the warmth of the water on your stomach ... your chest ... your back ... your arms ... your hands. You feel yourself becoming more still ... more peaceful inside ... you feel yourself quieting. You take another deep breath ... now imagine that you have a warm washcloth over your eyes ... the warmth of the washcloth gently soothes your eyelids ... now your jaws part and there is a little space between the roof of your mouth and your tongue ... you feel very, very relaxed....
>
> I'd now like for you to imagine, as you lie in this warm tub, a beautiful beach ... like you are looking at a snapshot. With your eyes closed, you see the clear blue of the sky ... the fluffy white clouds ... the sparkling sand ... you feel the soft wind as it blows in from the ocean and touches your face ... you feel the warmth of the sun as it gently shines down on your shoulders and hair ... you feel the soft sand beneath your feet ... you hear the sound of the waves as they roll into the shore ... you hear the sound of the wind ... the sound of seagulls in the distance ... you taste a little bit of the salt from the sea as it is carried in on the ocean breeze ... you smell the freshness of the sea and the warm baked smell of the sand ... you feel very much a part of all of this ... you feel very safe ... and relaxed ... and at peace.
>
> Know that at any time ... you can come back to this beautiful beach ... just by closing your eyes and breathing deeply.... I am now going to slowly count back from five to one ... with each number, you become more aware of being back in this room ... with all of the sounds outside ... all of your thoughts ... but you feel very unaffected by everything around you ... nothing can disturb this peace you have inside ... unless you choose to allow it to....
>
> Five ... you begin to become more aware of the sounds outside ... you turn your head from side to side and stretch a little.... Four ... remember that you

can go back to the beach and to this wonderful state of relaxation at any time you want to. . . . Three. . . . Two . . . and. . . . One . . . very, very slowly, take your time, you can come back into the room and open your eyes . . . feeling more relaxed and peaceful.

Ask your patients to rate their level of stress/anxiety/distress as soon as they open their eyes. Make sure you speak very softly and gently at first to allow them to slowly come back into the room. Most patients will report a lessening of distress after participating in this exercise. If not, find out what obstacles the patients experienced and let them know that, with practice, they will have greater success in using this strategy. Prescribe homework: breathing exercise (10 breaths) three times a day and relaxation (5 to 8 minutes) three times a week. Tell patients to practice the relaxation exercise when they are *not* very stressed, because, when learning a new technique, it is best to do it when there is more chance of success.

One final word about the relaxation/imagery exercise: reading the script to the patient is a nice way to become more comfortable with administering this intervention; however, you can also make an audiotape (using the provided script or one of your own) to be played while the patient is in the room.

Motivational Interviewing Strategies

A primary aim of MI is to assist the patient in moving from one stage of change to the next. Motivational interviewing interventions can be easily integrated into CBT visits. To find out where your patients are in the stages of change, a useful question to ask is, "How has your drinking and/or other drug use affected your life?" Precontemplators might answer, "Not at all. I've got it under control." Contemplators may respond with something to the effect of, "Well, sometimes I kind of go off the deep end, but, in general, it's not really a problem." Preparing patients might respond with, "Really bad, and I know I need to do something about it. I know I need help." Action patients might say, "It's affected my life so much that I had to stop." Maintainers might respond, "It affected me so much that I had to quit—it's been over 6 months now since I have had a drink or drug." Relapsers might reply, "It affected me a lot and so I stopped, but then I went back after awhile."

After identifying what stage your patient is in, you can then weave in the following stage-appropriate strategies (based on Miller's protocol [18]), into your first three visits, while you are also teaching the patient cognitive restructuring, mindfulness, and breathing/relaxation.

Strategies for Precontemplators

- Establish rapport, ask permission to discuss substance use, and build trust.
- Raise doubts or concerns in the patient about substance-using patterns by

- ○ Eliciting the patient's perception of the problem
- ○ Offering factual information about the risks of substance use
- ○ Exploring the pros and cons of substance use
- ○ Examining discrepancies between the patient's and others' perceptions of the problem behavior
- Express concern and keep the door open.

Strategies for Contemplators

- Normalize ambivalence. ("It's common to feel torn when you are thinking about the pros and cons of using. The [alcohol/drug] has been your friend for a long time, and it's probably hard to imagine not using any more.")
- Help your patient "tip the decisional balance scales" by
  - ○ Eliciting pros and cons of substance use and change (Figure 5.2 presents a Decision Balance handout to give your patients to aid with this goal)
  - ○ Examining the patient's personal values in relation to change (wise talk vs. the monkey)
  - ○ Emphasizing the patient's free choice, responsibility, and self-efficacy (their self-assessment of their perceived abilities/capacity) for change ("If you decided to stop using, it would totally be your choice and your responsibility—even though I would be here with you all the way. Do you feel that, if you wanted to stop using, you would be able to do it? What are some obstacles that might get in the way?")
  - ○ Eliciting self-motivational statements of intent and commitment from the patient and summarize them ("What can you tell yourself to motivate you or to help you feel more committed to wanting to change?" "Okay—so you say that if you stopped using you would feel happier, have a better life, and no longer fight with your wife. Is this accurate?")

Strategies for Preparators

- Clarify the patient's own goals and strategies for change.
- Offer a menu of options for change or treatment.
- With permission, offer expertise and advice.
- Negotiate a "change plan." ("Okay, I hear you saying you want to stop using by the end of the week and that you will go into detox on Friday afternoon. Is this right? Let's then make the agreement that you will do this and, after (or during) detox, you will call me to let me know how you are doing and also to schedule your next appointment with me so we can celebrate your success together. Does that sound like a good plan?")
- Consider and lower barriers to change. ("Let's try to look at any barriers that might get in your way to make you less likely to go into detox on Friday, and then we'll figure out how to get rid of them so you will definitely make it there as we have planned.")

You have a habit that is unhealthy. It has been pointed out that you should change this habit, but the decision is up to you. Before you can make the final decision to change or not to change, you need to consider all the risks and benefits to your decision. Please complete the following chart.

Considering Change	Reasons to Stay the Same	Reasons to Change
If _____ *Write in the unhealthy habit* **Stays the Same**	**Benefits** What do you like about.........?	**Concerns** What concerns you about.........?
If It Is Changed _____ *Write in a Goal for Change*	**Concerns** What concerns would you have about change?	**Benefits** What are the benefits of change?

Figure 5.2. Botelho's decision balance chart. (Courtesy of Rick Botelho, B Med Sci, University of Rochester, Rochester, NY.)

- Assist the patient to negotiate finances, child care, work, transportation, or other potential barriers.
- Help the patient enlist social support. ("Who can we ask to help support you during this time, just in case the monkey starts messing with you on Friday? Is there someone who is a positive support (who doesn't use) who can take you to detox?")
- Explore treatment (or Alcoholics Anonymous [AA], Narcotics Anonymous [NA] attendance if the patient does not need detox or inpatient/outpatient treatment) expectancies. ("Is there anything you are worried

about at the detox/treatment center/AA or NA meetings? What do you expect will happen there?")

- Elicit from the patient what has worked in the past for him or her or for someone else.
- Suggest that the patient publicly announce (to family, friends, possibly employer) plans to change.

Strategies for Action Patients

- Reinforce the importance of remaining in recovery.
- Support a realistic view of change through small steps (e.g., "one day at a time")
- Acknowledge difficulties for the patient in the early stages of change.
- Help the patient identify high-risk situations (e.g., going to a bar to hear a band, attending a wedding where alcohol will be served, etc.) and develop appropriate strategies to overcome these. ("I know you are upset and angry that you know you probably can't attend the wedding but— this is only temporary. After you get some time, some sobriety under your belt, you'll be able to go to all of the weddings you want.")
- Assist the patient in finding new reinforcers of positive change. ("Now you can go running and play with your kids without being exhausted or hung over. Also, it seems like you've made some really great friends at AA—why don't you go out with them after a meeting to have coffee or dinner?")

Strategies for Maintainers

- Continue to help the patient identify and sample drug-free sources of pleasure (i.e., new reinforcers).
- Support lifestyle changes. ("I know it cost a lot to move, but it was so worth it. Now you are away from the old neighborhood and you can start fresh—no one will be knocking at your door at 3 am to sell you some crack.")
- Affirm the patient's resolve and self-efficacy. ("I am so proud of you— you have done a really difficult thing. See, you are so much stronger and more courageous than you had thought you were. Your wise self *really* wants you to live and to have peace. Great job.")
- Help the patient practice and use new coping strategies to avoid a return to use.
- Maintain supportive contact (e.g., explain to the patient that you are available to talk between visits).
- Develop a "fire escape" plan if the patient returns to use. ("You are doing great right now, and I believe you will continue to do so. However, it is always good to have a 'fire escape' plan about what to do if you were to start sliding back into the 'fire' of alcohol/other drug use. For instance, the plan could be that no matter what, you agree to call me—even if your monkey is really loud [which it will be]—and you agree to come into the office immediately. What do you think about this?")
- Review long-term goals with the patient.

Strategies for the Patient Who Has Relapsed

- Help the patient reenter the change cycle and commend any willingness to reconsider positive change. ("Lots of people relapse, but not a lot of people come to their doctor and admit that they have relapsed. It's important to forgive yourself and to focus once again on today. Remember, the monkey wants you to feel a lot of guilt and shame because then you'll use again. What would your wise (God, Jehovah, Higher Power) self say to you right now to give you encouragement?")
- Explore the meaning and reality of the relapse as a learning opportunity (be positive and encouraging).
- Assist the patient in finding alternative coping strategies. ("So, you said you picked up a drink because you were angry with your wife. If you could go back, what could you have done differently, instead of picking up that drink, to deal with your anger?")
- Maintain supportive contact.

How to Implement Brief Cognitive-Behavioral Therapy and Motivational Interviewing Strategies in Your Practice

Once you are comfortable with assessing where a patient is in the stages of change, using stage-appropriate strategies, and teaching patients the CBT techniques of cognitive restructuring, mindfulness, and breathing/relaxation, the next question may be, "Okay, so how do I actually implement these things in my practice?" The easiest way to start may be to schedule weekly or biweekly (depending on your clinic schedule and patient caseload) 30- to 40-minute "stress management" or "behavioral follow-up" visits with your patients. These sessions, usually no more than three, are solely devoted to teaching patients aspects of CBT from an MI stages of change perspective. After these "teaching" visits, patients return once a month or so as needed for ongoing reinforcement of the concepts. In general, and in our experience, most patients (excluding patients with severe Axis I and/or personality disordered patients) usually need to return for only about four to five monthly behavioral follow-ups after the three teaching visits. Some patients will want to continue attending "booster sessions" once every 3 to 6 months after that. Of course, Precontemplators and Contemplators may need more visits (although they will not think so), and Action and Maintaining patients may need fewer. The key will be to be flexible and to operate from a patient-oriented perspective—the patient's progress will let you know just how much support he or she will need. A summary of the CBT and MI interventions for visits 1 to 3 are presented in Table 5.2.

Coding for these visits may be different depending on which state you are practicing in and which insurance carrier you are dealing with. The following "tips" generally apply for coding outpatient counseling: (1) If counseling is problem oriented and takes up more than 50% of face-to-face time, use E/M codes (99201–99215), with the chief complaint being medical/surgical in nature (e.g., fatigue, pain, insomnia); and (2) if counseling is preventative in nature, use a preventative code (99401–99404). In some states, psychotherapy codes (90804–90857) can be used by physicians who are not psychiatrists (25).

Table 5.2. Summary of cognitive-behavioral therapy and motivational interviewing strategies.

Visit one
- Ask "How has your drinking/drug use affected your life?" to assess stage of change. Use stage-appropriate strategies
- Teach patient that "we feel what we think" and how feelings influence physical sensations and behaviors
- Teach patient that the only thing he or she has control over is what is between his or her ears
- Teach patient about the monkey and the wise self
- Ask, "What can you tell yourself that would make you feel less _____ ?" or "What would (God or the wise part of you) tell you right now about the situation?"
- Suggested homework
  - Become aware of the monkey (negative self-talk)
  - Make a decision to change monkey talk to (God, wise self) talk
  - Live one day at a time

Visit two
- Ask patient about homework from first visit: successes in using cognitive restructuring and focusing on one day at a time? Obstacles or difficulties?
- Teach patient mindfulness (awareness) exercise as a way to "disconnect" from the monkey
- Continue to use strategies appropriate for patient's stage of change
- Suggested homework
  - Continue to be aware of how thoughts create feelings and make decision to change thoughts to change feelings
  - Practice mindfulness (awareness) exercise three times a day (10–15 seconds each time)

Visit three
- Ask patient about homework from last visit: Practice mindfulness/awareness exercise? Successes using this exercise? Obstacles or difficulties?
- Teach patient diaphragmatic breathing
- Teach patient brief relaxation/imagery exercise
- Continue to use strategies appropriate for patient's stage of change
- Suggested homework
  - Continue to be aware of how thoughts create feelings and make decision to change thoughts to change feelings
  - Practice diaphragmatic breathing three times a day (10 deep breaths each time)
  - Practice relaxation/imagery at least three times a week

In addition, the American Academy of Family Physicians offers the following tips for coding counseling visits: E/M services can be coded based on the time spent counseling the patient when that time constitutes more than 50% of the encounter (i.e., more than 50% of the face-to-face time you spend with the patient in the office or other outpatient setting or more than 50% of the floor/unit time you spend in the facility setting). To choose the correct Current Procedural Terminology code, compare the total time spent with the patient with the typical times listed in the code. For example, if you spend 15 minutes of a 25-minute office visit counseling an established patient, you could code that service 99214, because the total time spent with the patient (25 minutes) meets or exceeds the typical time listed for Current Procedural Terminology code 99214 (26).

Documentation of these visits should include a description of the counseling provided and the total length of the visit. It should also specify that over half of the time was spent in counseling to make it clear that you are coding the encounter based on time rather than on other key components (e.g., history, examination, medical decision making; for more information on time-based coding, see Sophocles [26]).

General Guidelines for Leading a Family Conference

Addiction is often characterized as a family disease, because it affects all individuals in the family unit. Hence, you may want to invite the patient, as well as his or her family members, into your office for a "family conference" (in addition to referring them for ongoing family therapy). The following are some general guidelines for leading a family conference in the primary care setting (for more information, see McDaniel et al. [27]).

- Normalize the artificiality of the situation and probable intensity of the underlying feelings of those present. ("You may find this a bit awkward, all of us meeting here to talk about how Joe's drinking has affected the entire family. There are probably a lot of feelings—anger, fear, sadness—that each of you has.")
- Immediately set boundaries with all present. This might include your expectations regarding participation, such as speaking one at a time without interrupting, no name-calling, or screaming and acknowledging the limited time of the visit. Have everyone present agree to follow these boundaries. ("We only have thirty minutes, so we will start by having each family member talk about his or her feelings about Joe's drinking for 5 minutes each [longer if only one or two family members present; adjust time accordingly with the understanding that there will probably never be enough time—these family members have likely been holding in their feelings for years], and then we will ask Joe to comment on what he has heard.")
- Establish goals for today's visit. ("We are here today to figure out how to best help Joe stop drinking and to figure out how each of you can take care of yourselves during this process.")

- Ask each family member to tell Joe what his or her concerns are about Joe's drinking (or how his drinking has affected that member) for the previously agreed on length of time. Be aware that anger may surface. Validate anger (or whatever emotion the family member is expressing), but redirect if anger starts to escalate. ("Lori, I know how angry you must be right now and how difficult this must be to be telling Joe all of these things. I am sure you are reliving them in your mind right now. But let's try to remember that we are here—and Joe is here—to work on stopping his alcohol use. If you can, try to 'report' to him how you are feeling without actually losing yourself in your anger right now. Is that okay? Your anger is valid and normal and should be expressed in an appropriate place—that is why I am also referring you all to family therapy.")
- After each family member participates, ask Joe to summarize what he heard and to say how he thinks his drinking has affected him and his family. Ask him to set a goal.
- Refer Joe to AA (or detox first if needed) and the family to Al-Anon. Encourage each person to focus only on what he or she has to do for himself or herself. ("Lori, it is important that you let Joe go to his AA meetings and that you focus on Al-Anon for you. The kids should go to Ala-Teen. You may be tempted, as Joe might, to ask each other what happened at the meeting the other attended or whether or not the other is attending meetings regularly. I am going to suggest that you take the focus off each other and only think about what you need to do—not what the other needs to do—for your own recovery.")
- Refer the family to family therapy but also offer to see them for regular (monthly, bimonthly, etc.) conferences in your office if needed. However, always ask what is happening in family therapy, and build on it in your visits (you do not want to suggest strategies that might be in opposition to what they are learning in regular therapy). Obtain a release of information so that you can speak to the therapist as needed.

References

1. Hester RK, Squires DD. Outcome research: alcoholism. In Galanter M, Kleber HD, eds. Textbook of Substance Abuse Treatment. Arlington, VA: American Psychiatric Association; 2004;129–135.
2. Parsons JT, Rosof E, Punzalan JC, DiMaria L. Integration of motivational interviewing and cognitive behavioral therapy to improve HIV medication adherence and reduce substance use among HIV-positive men and women: results of a pilot project. AIDS Patient Care STDS 200519:31–39.
3. Baker A, Lee NK, Claire M, Lewin TJ, Grant T, Pohlman S, Saunders JB, Kay-Lambkin F, Constable P, Jenner L, Carr VJ. Brief cognitive behavioural interventions for regular amphetamine users: a step in the right direction. Addiction 2005;100(3):367–378.

4. Bertholet N, Daeppen J-B, Wietlisbach V, Fleming M, Burnand B. Reduction of alcohol consumption by brief alcohol intervention in primary care: systematic review and meta-analysis. Arch Intern Med 2005;165:986–995.

5. Beck AT. A systematic investigation of depression. Compr Psychiatry 1961;2: 162–170.

6. Beck AT. Thinking and depression. Arch Gen Psychiatry 1963;9:324–333.

7. Beck AT. Depression. New York: Hoeber-Harper; 1967.

8. Beck A, Weisharr M. Cognitive therapy. In Freeman A, Simon KM, Butler LE, Arkowitz H, eds. Comprehensive Handbook of Cognitive Therapy. New York: Plenum Press; 1989.

9. Ellis A. Group rational-emotive and cognitive-behavioral therapy. Int J Group Psychother 1992;42(1):63–80.

10. Persons JB. Cognitive Therapy in Practice: A Case Formulation Approach. New York: W.W. Norton & Company, 1989.

11. Botelho RJ, Novak S. Dealing with substance misuse, abuse, and dependency. Primary Care 1993;20(1):51–70.

12. Bien TH, Miller WR, Tonigan JS. Brief interventions for alcohol problems: a review. Addiction 1993;88(3):315–335.

13. Haynes P, Ayliffe G. Locus of control of behaviour: is high externality associated with substance misuse? Br J Addict 1991;86(9):1111–1117.

14. Rollnick S, Heather N, Gold R, Hall W. Development of a short "readiness to change" questionnaire for use in brief, opportunistic interventions among excessive drinkers. Br J Addict 1992;87(5):743–754.

15. Secades-Villa R, Fernande-Hermida JR, Arnaez-Montaraz C. Motivational interviewing and treatment retention among drug user patients: a pilot study. Subst Use Misuse 2004;39(9):1369–1378.

16. Stotts AL, Schmitz JM, Rhoades HM, Grabowski J. Motivational interviewing with cocaine-dependent patients: a pilot study. J Consult Clin Psychol 2001;69(5): 858–862.

17. Prochaska JO, DiClemente CC. The Transtheoretical Approach: Crossing Traditional Boundaries of Therapy. Homewood, IL: Dow Jones-Irwin; 1984.

18. Miller WR. Enhancing Motivation for Change in Substance Abuse Treatment. Treatment Improvement Protocol (TIP) Series (35) 1999. Rockville, MD: U.S. Department of Health and Human Services.

19. DiClemente CC, Prochaska JO, Fairhurst SK, Velicer WF, Velasquez MM, Rossi JS. The process of smoking cessation: an analysis of precontemplation, contemplation, and preparation stages of change. J Consult Clin Psychol. 1991;59(2):295–304.

20. Marlatt GA, Gordon JR, eds. Relapse Prevention: Maintenance Strategies in the Treatment of Addictive Behaviors. New York: Guilford Press; 1985.

21. Pattison M. Finding peace and joy in the practice of medicine. Health Prog 2006;87(3):22.

22. Puchalski C. Spirituality in health: the role of spirituality in critical care. Crit Care Clin 2004;20(3):487–504.

23. Bennett M. Spirituality and addictions. What do we know? Addictions Newslett 1998;6:5–26.
24. Carter JH. Religion/spirituality in African-American culture: an essential aspect of psychiatric care. J Natl Med Assoc 2002;94:371–375.
25. Weinman HM. Doc-U-Tips. Baptist Health/Baptist Medical Center, September 2005. Available at: execdoc@aol.com.
26. Sophocles A. Time is of the essence: coding on the basis of time for physician services. Family Practice Management, June 2003:27. Available at: http://www.aafp.org/fpm/20030600/27time.html.
27. McDaniel SH, Campbell TL, Hepworth J, Lorenz A, Satcher D. Family-Oriented Primary Care: A Manual for Medical Providers. New York, Springer; 2005.

6. Case Presentations and Algorithms for Management

The case presentations in this chapter illustrate three types of patients who are frequently seen in the primary care setting. Each case is followed by an algorithm based on recommendations discussed in previous chapters. It is our hope that the material presented thus far will provide clarity into how to manage each case.

Case 1: Linda

Presentation

Linda is a 44-year-old white woman who, when you see her name on your schedule, causes you to cringe and hope that she is a no-show for her appointment. However, you know your wish is in vain: Linda *always* shows up. She never fails to complain of a new, acute event occurring in her life: the breakup of a relationship, problems at work, issues with money and/or the kids. The only consistent, predictable thing in Linda's life, it seems, is the answer to all of her problems—Xanax—and she will not consider any of the other pharmacologic or nonpharmacologic strategies you have suggested.

On Monday, Linda comes in for her appointment. As usual, there are new crises in her life: her car broke down and her eldest son was arrested for shoplifting. Not that this isn't bad enough, Linda informs you that the medication is no longer effective at the present dosage, and, in fact, she has taken matters into her own hands by doubling the dosage. Of course, she has now run out of her prescription and needs you to give her a refill. Realizing the dangers of withdrawal by not refilling her prescription at the present dosage, you feel that she has you "up against the wall" and, understandably, you feel very angry and frustrated. However, being the prudent physician you are, you attempt to regain control of the situation by telling her that you are going to limit her refill and give her another appointment later that same week to "sit down and talk about other options we can come up with to manage your anxiety—after this point in time, Xanax is potentially hurting, more than helping, you." Linda agrees and thanks you profusely as you write her refill (enough for the next 3 days). When Thursday comes, Linda does not show up for her appointment. Late in the afternoon on Friday, she calls—apologizing that yet another crisis (her employer threatened to fire her) caused her to miss her appointment yesterday. In fact, she informs you that she took "two extra doses" of Xanax to help "calm me down because he upset me so much," and she ran out of her medication this morning. She goes on to inform you that she presently feels "sweaty" and that "my heart is racing and it feels like it's going to jump out of my chest." Linda further reports that her anxiety is 12 on a scale of 10.

Discussion

A. Inform Linda that she needs to come in immediately or go to the emergency room. Inform her that she is in danger of withdrawal and that withdrawal from Xanax can be fatal. Also let her know that you can no longer prescribe for her if she does not come in to see you, as doing so would be harmful to her health (document your recommendations and her response). If she does come back to see you, the following is suggested:

1. Physical examination: Obtain a complete physical examination if one has not been done recently.
2. Perform a comprehensive substance use/abuse history:
   a. Go over each substance type, including amount, frequency, and for how long it has been used. Be certain to include an alcohol use history!
   b. Determine whether she meets the criteria for substance dependence.
   c. Determine whether she has an anxiety disorder. If so, did her anxiety symptoms begin prior to her substance use? (Differentiate whether dependence is a primary disorder and not the result of an anxiety disorder [see (d) below] or whether she has both disorders, i.e., substance dependence co-occurring with an anxiety disorder.)
   d. Attempt to ascertain whether dependence is iatrogenic (i.e., patient had an anxiety disorder but tolerance to Xanax got out of control. In other words, she does not have addictive illness [i.e., a substance use disorder] but, rather, in our experience, she is exhibiting symptoms similar to the definition of "pseudoaddiction" discussed in Chapter 1.)
3. Obtain laboratory work:
   a. Make sure that a complete blood count (CBC) with differential and liver function tests (LFTs) are included. You will be looking for mean corpuscular volume (MCV) and gamma-glutamyl transpeptidase (GGT) elevations (elevations show alcohol effect). Alcohol is often abused with benzodiazepines.
   b. Include a urine drug screen (UDS). Specifically ask for a complete benzodiazepine panel as part of this screen. If you are suspicious of opioid use (from the history), be certain that the drug screen includes a screen for synthetic opioid medications.
4. Refer the patient to an inpatient detoxification facility: Referral is indicated because the home situation is not stable and recent

behaviors (losing prescriptions, running out of medication, not keeping her appointments) suggest that this patient is not a good candidate for outpatient detox. If withdrawal symptoms have become too problematic by the time she arrives, referral to detox might be the only thing you do for this visit.

5. If the patient has an underlying anxiety disorder (determined by history), we again recommend inpatient detoxification, but discuss with the treatment provider the use of a low dose of a selective serotonin uptake inhibitor (SSRI) to begin either during detox or early in the treatment after detox.

B. If the patient does not have the means to pay for detox and a publicly funded (indigent) detox is not available in your area, then be prepared to follow up with the patient and provide outpatient detox (via Klonopin for no more than 2 to 4 weeks) *with a strict contract/agreement* (which will include participation in 12 Step meetings, obtaining a 12 Step sponsor, etc.; see Medication Management Agreement in Appendix 2).

1. If you will be managing her detox, begin a low dose of an SSRI at the beginning of the detox period (do not titrate until after detox is complete). This step is necessary if she has a comorbid anxiety/substance dependence problem and can be skipped if there is no evidence of an anxiety disorder.

2. Note that post-acute withdrawal syndrome can mimic an anxiety disorder (sleep disturbance, increased anxiety and worry, etc.), but these symptoms will decrease over a several-month period. The symptoms of an anxiety disorder will not decrease over time.

3. After completion of the detox protocol (Klonopin, no more than 2 to 4 weeks), *do not restart benzodiazepines at any time!* Encourage the patient to increase attendance at 12 Step meetings, meet regularly with her sponsor, and other positive supports. Use the stages of change and cognitive-behavioral therapy (CBT) strategies to assist her in gaining more control over her distressful feelings.

4. If the patient turns out to have only an anxiety disorder and not a comorbid diagnosis of substance dependence (i.e., she is a "pseudo-addict" not a "true" addict), you may consider the following:

   a. Take the maximum dosage of Xanax that she has used, convert it to Klonopin using an approximate 1:1 ratio, and divide it into four times a day dosing for approximately 2 days (looking for remission of withdrawal symptoms and no drowsiness). Titrate to stability as necessary; and maintain for approximately 2 days.

   b. Start an SSRI after she is stable on Klonopin.

   c. After she is stable, begin a very slow Klonopin wean (weeks to months).

   d. Use a very strict benzodiazepine agreement/contract.

   e. Maintain urine drug screens on a random (but regularly performed) basis. Because she should not drink during this phase, if she can afford it, we recommend intermittent ethyl glucuronide (ETG) testing in place of the routine drug screens.

f. Titration decisions regarding the SSRI can be difficult, as side effects can mimic withdrawal symptoms; therefore, proceed with caution and consultation when necessary.

Case 2: Bill

Presentation

Bill is a 52-year-old African-American man who has been your patient for many years. He is the chief executive officer of a local, successful business, and he had always been very active in the community. Over the years, he had been on numerous boards and involved in outreach programs. You attend the same church as Bill, and you had been seeing him there on a regular basis. Historically, he had been diligent about coming in for his routine examinations, but you have noticed that, for the past couple of years, he has not scheduled an appointment. In fact, upon noticing this, you also realize that you have not seen him in church for a very long time. You decide to give him a call to see how he is doing. Bill sounds almost too cheerful as he informs you that he has not been in because he has been "too busy." This perplexes you somewhat, because you know how active Bill had always been in his health care—in addition to regularly attending his appointments for routine examinations, he was also very involved in running and in working out at the local YMCA. When you suggest that he come in for a physical, Bill agrees.

Bill arrives late for his appointment. During the examination, you find that he has lost 10 pounds since his last examination 2 years ago. Bill informs you that he has stopped running because "my work schedule has been too crazy." His blood pressure is mildly elevated, as is his GGT. Upon questioning, you find that Bill's life appears rather chaotic and stressful. He reports that his marriage has "gone to hell" and, specifically, he tells you that his wife, Rebecca, "nags me all the time" and that she "sure as hell isn't the sweet girl I married!" Because of Bill's laboratory results, weight loss, and blood pressure, you ask him about any changes in alcohol use. Bill laughs loudly and shrugs, stating, "No, Doc. I just have a couple of drinks once a week or so—you would too if you were married to my wife!" He then proceeds to discuss his dissatisfaction with his marriage. At the end of the visit, Bill agrees to go back to exercising, decrease his salt intake, and resume his previous diet of eating three healthful meals a day—no matter how "crazy" his work schedule becomes. He additionally agrees to return for follow-up in 3 months to recheck his liver enzymes and blood pressure. You also recommend a good family therapist and invite Bill to bring his wife in to meet you for a family conference, if he so wishes.

Two weeks after his appointment with you, you notice in the local newspaper that Bill had been arrested for driving under the influence. In fact, the day you read the story, you also receive a call from Rebecca, Bill's wife. She tells you that she is "really worried" about Bill because "he drinks every day and it causes him to have mood swings." You ask Rebecca to please tell Bill to call you, but Bill does not call. A week later, his wife contacts you again, very agitated, to inform you that Bill is "sweating a lot" and has chest pain. You instruct Rebecca to take Bill to the nearest emergency room immediately (or call 911). Later that day, the emergency room physician calls you to inform you that Bill's electrocardiogram and other cardiac tests were all normal but that his alanine aminotransferase level is significantly elevated, his MCV is mildly elevated, and his blood pressure is "sky high." He goes on to state that he suspects alcohol withdrawal and he has admitted Bill into the hospital.

You decide to go visit Bill. When you arrive, Rebecca is also present in the room. Bill appears "dopey" but stable. Upon questioning, you discover that Bill had made a "deal" with his wife. Rather than go to couples' counseling with the family therapist you had recommended, he suggested that they go away for an "alcohol-free" weekend. Because of bad weather, the drive home had taken much longer than originally anticipated and Bill's symptoms grew progressively worse.

When you ask Bill directly about his drinking and whether or not he thinks he might have a problem, he waves his hands and remarks loudly, "Doc, you sound just like my wife! Let me tell you what I told her—I can quit whenever I want to. See? I went the whole weekend without a *drop!* Maybe I had been drinking a little too much lately. My job is very stressful. Maybe I'll go ahead and cut back a little bit."

Discussion

A. Identify which stage of change Bill is in ("How has drinking affected your life, Bill?"), and use clinical strategies for that stage.
B. Schedule him for a follow-up visit in your office immediately after discharge from the hospital. However, the preference is either have the hospital perform the detox or refer him directly to a detox program from the hospital.
C. If he has not been detoxed and has an appointment in your office, obtain the results of the physical examination and laboratory tests performed in the hospital
   1. Obtain a substance abuse history and UDS.
   2. If Bill seems to be in the Preparation stage (i.e., ready to commit to time to start a plan to get sober):
      a. Refer him to inpatient detox if his last drink was less than 4 to 5 days ago.
      b. After he is discharged from detox and comes back to see you in your office (or as soon as possible if he does not need detox), teach Bill CBT techniques and use strategies for patients in the Action stage (if he is still not drinking after detox).
      c. Recommend outpatient treatment (if the detox facility has not already made this recommendation).

    d. If Bill is fearful of a relapse and requests pharmacologic support until he is enrolled into outpatient treatment, start naltrexone and/or acamprosate.
    e. Obtain a release of information so you can speak with the outpatient treatment providers.
    f. Recommend Alcoholics Anonymous (AA) and getting a sponsor.
    g. Recommend Al-Anon for his wife and other interested family members.
3. If Bill appears to be in the Precontemplation or Contemplation stage:
    a. Refer him for inpatient detox, as above.
    b. Attempt to help him realize the need for inpatient treatment; however, if he refuses, strongly recommend outpatient treatment.
        i. Follow up with Antabuse or naltrexone and/or acamprosate as indicated.
        ii. Follow up with random UDS, including ETG.
        iii. Perform follow-up laboratory tests (CBC, LFTs) every 3 months.
        iv. Recommend AA and getting a sponsor.
        v. Recommend Al-Anon for his wife and other interested family members.
4. Note that because of being in either Precontemplation or Contemplation, Bill may not seek treatment—even with your strong recommendation—at this time. Teach Bill CBT techniques and use strategies for Precontemplators or Contemplators in the hope that he will eventually move toward Action. You might also consider entering into an agreement with him that he will go to treatment if he cannot "stay stopped."

Case 3: Lucy

Presentation

Lucy is a 24-year-old white woman who is single and who has two children, ages 3 and 5 years. She is a new patient, and her only insurance is Medicaid. She presents with chronic low back pain, which she states began after the birth of her second child. She claims to be unable to work secondary to her pain, which she describes as "sharp" and rates its intensity as 9 on a scale of 10. Upon initial observation, you note no abnormalities in gait or difficulties in changing positions. Of interest, you also note that she grimaces only when asked specific questions about her pain. Historically, you can elicit no evidence of acute trauma subsequent to her last childbirth. During her physical, you note no neurologic deficits or any other positive physical symptoms, including complaints of radiculopathy.

At the conclusion of this first visit, Lucy asks for pain medication. She states that she has seen numerous doctors before you and has made several visits to the emergency room, but only "certain" medications have helped. She informs you that she is allergic to codeine and that Darvocet has "never worked." When you propose the idea to initiate an antiinflammatory, she quickly informs you that she has "tried them all and none of them work." She then tells you what *does* work: "Lortab or Vicodin and Soma." In fact, during acute exacerbation of her pain, she also finds the addition of Xanax to be "very useful." She further informs you that she "ran out of my medications yesterday." You write prescriptions (reluctantly and against your better judgment) for 2 weeks of Lorcet and Soma and you also send her for blood work and magnetic resonance imaging (MRI). When you suggest referral to a local pain clinic, Lucy quickly informs you that "it's too much money and they don't take Medicaid."

One week later, you receive a phone call from Lucy. She sounds frantic and demanding. She informs you that she is in "excruciating" pain and she has run out of her medication. When asked, she tells you she has not had a chance to schedule the MRI because both of her kids have been sick. She has had the laboratory work done, but your office has not yet received the results. You tell Lucy to go to the emergency room and then to call the office for a follow-up visit. You see her 3 days later in your office. She was given Demerol intramuscularly and Ativan by mouth in the emergency room and discharged with 3 days of Lorcet and Soma. By the time of her appointment with you, she is out of all of her medications. Upon looking at the chart, you realize she had finished your original 2-week prescriptions in 1 week. Despite this, along with the recent emergency room prescriptions, she still complains of severe pain and insomnia. She also states that she "can't take care of my kids and they still have colds" while she is in pain and she is not getting any sleep. You notice in her chart that the laboratory results have come back and that they are all within normal range.

Discussion

A. Perform a physical examination if one has not been performed recently.
B. Perform a comprehensive substance use/abuse history. Again, as with Linda, be certain to go over each substance type, including amount, frequency, and for how long it was used. Include an alcohol use history.
C. Obtain laboratory tests (specifically the following if not in the chart):
   1. Be certain to include a CBC with differential and LFTs. You will be looking for MCV and GGT elevations (indicating an alcohol effect).
   2. Obtain a UDS. Include a benzodiazepine panel that tests for all benzodiazepines, including Xanax, Ativan, and Klonopin. In addition, be certain that the opiates tested for include synthetics.
D. Obtain a release of information from Lucy's prior physicians, including workup results. This will probably take some time, and you cannot wait to receive the information before initiating a treatment plan. This patient and her family are in crisis!

E. Teach Lucy CBT strategies and assess where she is in the stages of change. Use clinical strategies appropriate for that stage.
F. Assess family support:
   1. If support is adequate, her family can care for the children while she enters inpatient detox followed by residential treatment.
   2. If there is no family support and the treatment facility has a mother–child residential program, refer to this program for detox and treatment
G. If neither of the above exists, this is a difficult situation. You might have no choice but to initiate outpatient detox via clonidine or baclofen. She will need to agree to a strict contract, with the threat to inform the state authorities if she does not comply. (Her children are in danger. Include in the contract an agreement that if she has a difficult time staying abstinent, she will go to an inpatient treatment setting. She should understand that you will not contact or involve child welfare authorities if she complies with this type of treatment, given that her children's welfare will be arranged.) With this approach, we would include outpatient treatment, Narcotics Anonymous, and obtaining a sponsor.
   1. Random, unscheduled UDSs are indicated. Include ETG, as total abstinence is required.
   2. Consider the need for naltrexone.
      a. Vivitrol is not yet indicated for opioid dependence, but is anticipated in the near future (possibly under another name).
      b. If Vivitrol is not available or feasible, Lucy can benefit from monitored intake of naltrexone three to five times per week (monitor her actual swallowing of the medication each time). If this is to be performed in your office, the nurse can administer from the patient's supply.
   3. Make sure that the UDS also tests for Xanax, Ativan, Klonopin, and synthetic opioids, including methadone.

Appendix 1. Into Action: Putting Cognitive-Behavioral Therapy and Motivational Interviewing into Practice

This appendix illustrates how the cognitive-behavioral and motivational strategies introduced in Chapter 5 can be put into practice. As previously discussed, you do not need to be a trained therapist to implement these strategies; many primary care physicians regularly counsel their patients using a variety of techniques. The following "transcript," which details a doctor–patient interaction over the course of three visits, is meant to assist you in gaining a clearer concept of how to use these interventions with your addicted patients. It is often said in the 12 Step programs to "take what you need and leave the rest." This is our recommendation to you too; use what interventions you feel comfortable with and either leave or change the rest to suit your own specific style and comfort level.

Visit One: Helping Your Patient Get the Monkey off Her Back

You have scheduled Linda to come back for a behavioral follow-up/stress management visit because you are greatly concerned about her Xanax use. The following is a script, using elements from both motivational interviewing (MI) and cognitive-behavioral therapy (CBT).

> **Doctor:** Linda, I asked you to come in today so we can talk about some of the stressors in your life. I like to see most of my patients for stress management visits, in addition to their regular medical visits. Everyone has stress, and I believe it's important to not only focus on the physical aspects of a person—it's important to also talk about one's thoughts, feelings, relationships, and sexual and spiritual aspects as well. Is this okay with you?
>
> **Linda:** Yes, I guess so.
>
> **Doctor:** I also need to let you know that this is *not* psychotherapy. However, if you and I feel that you might also benefit from traditional, weekly psychotherapy, I will give you some referrals, okay?
>
> **Linda:** That sounds okay.
>
> **Doctor:** Great! So, tell me, what is the biggest source of stress in your life right now? *(Note that the doctor does not immediately talk about the patient's drug use.)*

Linda: My anxiety. Also, my boyfriend just broke up with me.

Doctor: And you are sad about that.

Linda: Very! We were together a long time.

Doctor: Breakups are very difficult. After asking you a few more questions, I will teach you something that will help with those stressful feelings. *(Note that the doctor does not want to focus on Linda's relationship issues at the moment but reassures Linda that they will come back to this topic later.)*

Linda: Good. I need something to help me right now.

Doctor: Now that you mentioned that, I know you have used Xanax to help you when you've been under stress before. *(Note that the Doctor used Linda's words to segue into a discussion of her medication use.)*

Linda: (nods)

Doctor: Linda, how has your use of Xanax affected your life? *(MI question to assess which stage Linda is in.)*

Linda: Oh, the Xanax hasn't affected my life at all. It's my boyfriend that has really screwed things up! *(Her answer indicates that Linda is in the Precontemplative stage.)*

Doctor: I can see how frustrated you are. Linda, I would like to talk with you about your use of Xanax, if that's okay with you, because I am concerned. *(MI and strategies for Precontemplators: ask permission, express concern.)*

Linda: What are you concerned about? I don't have a problem with it.

Doctor: Linda, Xanax is a highly addictive drug. It has a very short half-life, meaning it does not stay in your system very long, and so often has interdose withdrawal, which means that your anxiety actually gets worse in between doses if you use this medication long term. Does that make sense to you?

Linda: Yes. I think I understand.

Doctor: Okay. Also, right after you take the Xanax, and other benzo-diazepines (which is the drug class that Xanax belongs to) the medication tends to knock out all anxiety—including *normal* anxiety—until the effects wear off and then your overall anxiety increases over time. Emotions such as anger, fear, sadness are not *bad*, they are totally normal feelings that we all have. For instance, if I didn't have fear, I would just walk across the street without looking both ways. And lots of positive things have happened in this world because good people got angry. We wouldn't have civil rights, equal rights, and lots of other important, positive changes if people had not gotten angry enough to lobby for these changes. Anger can be very productive and energizing! And, it's totally normal to feel sad or "blue" sometimes—especially when we have experienced a loss in our lives. It's just when these emotions get "stuck," and we feel them all the time ... *that's* when there is a problem. So, because the Xanax causes you to feel little to no anxiety when you have just taken it, you may feel that other nonaddictive medications (which are not in the same class as Xanax) aren't working when you try them because you are able to feel "normal" anxiety again. *(pauses)*

I have another thought about anxiety. I think that, at one time, it was a very healthy, positive thing to feel anxious much of the time, especially for women. What I mean is, back in the "old days," when a bear could burst through the window at any moment and steal your kids, it was a positive survival mechanism for the mother to be "on guard" most of the time. If she wasn't, one of her kids might wander off and get eaten by that bear! Not a great thought, but maybe the constant anxiety helped the mother protect her kids while the father was out gathering food. Although anxiety occurs in greater numbers among women, men have anxiety too, and that might also be related to their "guarding" role of days past. Maybe we used to be "guarders" and "gatherers" and this helped our species to survive. However, now the anxiety that has been passed along through generations of women and men isn't so positive or adaptive anymore. *(pauses)*

I've said a lot. Does this all make sense? Do you have any questions about anything I have just said? *(MI: provide factual information. Notice that the doctor does not directly confront the denial evident in her previous statement. The doctor discloses some of his own thoughts to assist the patient in understanding anxiety and to increase rapport. The doctor then checks the patient's understanding.)*

Linda: I didn't know any of that. About how maybe at one time, feeling anxious was a good thing. But it makes sense. I also didn't know about the Xanax creating more anxiety or about how it's normal to feel anxious sometimes.

Doctor: It's not very common knowledge. A lot of people do not know this. *(He normalizes Linda's lack of knowledge in this area.)* Linda, I have noticed that you frequently need to refill your prescription before it's due and that you are taking a lot more than we had initially agreed on. This tells me you probably have an incredible amount of stress your life, am I right? *(MI: build trust; gently confront.)*

Linda: Yes, always. I don't know what I would do without the Xanax. It's the only thing that helps me. *(In an indirect way, Linda may be telling the doctor that she is very afraid that she cannot live without her drug and that she may be terrified that he may be thinking about taking it away from her.)*

Doctor: Do you think that might be a problem? That you are very reliant on the medication? *(MI: elicit the patient's perspective on the problem.)*

Linda: Well, yeah, I guess. But don't some people just need to be on medication to cope? *(Linda is probably hoping that her doctor will just answer "yes" and not question her any further!)*

Doctor: Many people take medications to help them cope. But when the medication becomes the focus point, and it is taken in larger amounts than prescribed, this suggests that the person may have a problem with the medication and needs to learn more healthy types of coping strategies. I care about you, Linda, and want to help you feel better. I am on your side. *(MI: build trust.)*

Linda: I know you are. You have been a good doctor to me.

Doctor: Thank you, Linda. Tell you what: let's make an agreement from here on out. Let's agree that you will continue on the Xanax, at the dosage you are on right now, but that I will slowly reduce the dosage over time—after we have discussed this further. We will meet more regularly for this kind of visit. And I will use other medications, as well as teach you some alternative, healthy coping strategies, to deal with your anxiety that will be so much better for you over the long run than the Xanax. *(Many Precontemplators will not agree to this. However, Linda has a very good relationship with her doctor and may be open to this suggestion because she doesn't have to stop the medication right away. Please note: As the prescribing physician, you may have to make a firm call, even with Precontemplators, if you feel they are using their medications inappropriately. Some patients will need to be told that unless they agree to either decreasing their medications or having their medications prescribed by a psychiatrist, you may not be able to see them anymore.)*

Linda: So I won't have to stop the Xanax today?

Doctor: No. We'll go along on this dosage for awhile and then talk about reducing it slowly the next time we meet so you won't go into withdrawal, because withdrawal from this type of medication can be pretty dangerous. I am going to make sure that you are as comfortable as possible through this process. Never stop a drug you are taking without talking to me or another doctor first, okay? *(MI: provide factual information; build rapport. The doctor is also reassuring the patient about her fear of stopping the drug by letting her know he will keep her "comfortable.")*

Linda: (relieved) Okay. *(Now that Linda sees that the doctor is not planning to stop the medication immediately, she may be more open to what the doctor suggests.)*

Doctor: Great! Now I would like to teach you a very effective coping strategy. But first, let me ask you this: do you like animals? *(Changing focus, using humor.)*

Linda: (looking perplexed) Um, yes (smiles).

Doctor: Me, too! What is your favorite animal?

Linda: I really love dogs. I have two.

Doctor: I love dogs too. I also really like horses and dolphins, but I can't stand monkeys. You are probably wondering at this point why I am talking to you about animals and monkeys.

Linda: (nods and smiles)

Doctor: Well, after I am finished, you'll find out! Seriously, can you bear with me a moment? *(MI: ask permission.)*

Linda: (still smiling) Okay.

Doctor: So, I was talking about my dislike of monkeys. The reason that I don't like them is that they are loud, nasty, mean, and obscene! The problem is, we all have a monkey that lives inside our head. Now, it's not a *real* monkey, of course. It's the negative, ongoing chatter of our thoughts. *(CBT: introducing the concept of negative self-talk.)*

Linda: (nods in agreement)

Doctor: The most important thing I am going to say for the next few minutes is this: *we feel what we think,* or, whatever we think, we feel. The monkey is not our friend—it loves taking us into the future and to "what if"? Like, "what if" this bad thing happens, or "what if" this other bad thing happens. For example, your monkey sounds like it's been telling you, "what if my doctor stops the Xanax?" "What if I can't function without the medication and I fall apart?" "What if my anxiety gets worse?" "What if I never meet another guy and I am alone all of my life?" Do these thoughts sound familiar to you? *(CBT: introducing the link between thoughts and feelings.)*

Linda: Yes. It's as if you know exactly what I have been thinking! (smiles)

Doctor: Yes, I know your monkey, because I have one too! Actually, *everyone* has a monkey. When you are thinking "what if" thoughts like these, what are you feeling? *(CBT: teaching about thoughts creating feelings.)*

Linda: Scared. Nervous.

Doctor: Yes. Exactly. Remember, "*we feel what we think,*" so when you are thinking "what if" all of these bad things happen, you feel scared, nervous, very anxious. Good. Now, this monkey also loves to take us to the past to think about all of the "woulda, coulda, shouldas." If I go to the past and think about all of the mistakes I have made, all of the bad choices, all of the people who hurt me, I am going to feel depressed, guilty, ashamed, resentful. "If only I woulda done that" or "I shoulda done this." Do you see how these types of thoughts about the past create those distressful feelings? *(CBT: more teaching on the link between thoughts and feelings.)*

Linda: Yes. I do that all the time. But I think I worry more about the future.

Doctor: And that makes sense. You are more concerned with anxiety than with depression. Anxiety exists in the future, and depression tends to stem from past-oriented thoughts (although you can feel depressed about the future as well).

So, our thoughts create our feelings. Our feelings also affect our bodily sensations and our behaviors. For example, when you think about the future, you notice you feel anxious. How does that anxiety feel in your body? What bodily sensations do you have? *(CBT: introducing the thoughts, feelings, somatic sensations, behavior link.)*

Linda: My heart beats fast, and my hands get all clammy. I get a headache, too.

Doctor: You have very good insight and awareness of your bodily sensations. And when you are thinking about the future, feeling anxious, and your heart starts beating faster and your hands are clammy, what do you do? *(CBT: increasing patient's awareness of behaviors.)*

Linda: I take a Xanax.

Doctor: You are being very honest, and I really appreciate that. Taking medications like Xanax is what a lot of people want to do when they feel really anxious. Anxiety is *not* a comfortable feeling, is it? *(The doctor rewards her honesty with a very empathic, normalizing statement rather than scolding her for taking the medication.)*

Linda: No way!

Doctor: So, this is the bad news: We all have a monkey, and it always makes us feel bad when we listen to it. It is the part of us that is centered in fear and is totally irrational. As I said earlier, the monkey is not your friend! In fact, your monkey definitely does not want you to be talking to me right now because I care about you and I want to help you to feel better, to have more peace. Your monkey wants the opposite: It wants you to feel terrible. It wants you to be at home, alone, taking more and more Xanax. *(The doctor summarizes previous information about negative self-talk.)*

So, that's the bad news. The *good* news, however, is that we all have a part of us that is infinitely more powerful than the monkey could ever be. This is the part of you that wants peace, love, joy. This is the part of you that doesn't want to depend on any medication, the part of you that didn't run out the door when I told you that we would be decreasing your Xanax. Let me ask you a question: Do you believe in something bigger than yourself? *(CBT: introducing rational, balanced thinking and assessing spiritual beliefs.)*

Linda: Yes, I do.

Doctor: And what do you call it? *(MI: expressing interest in finding out what the patient thinks/believes.)*

Linda: I don't really have a name for it. I guess I think of it as my "Higher Power."

Doctor: Okay. Can I ask you a few questions about your Higher Power, because your idea of your Higher Power may be different from my idea of my Higher Power, and I want to make sure that we are using *your* belief, because that is what will be helpful to you. *(MI: building trust and rapport.)*

Linda: Sure.

Doctor: Okay. Is your Higher Power loving? Does it love you?

Linda: Yes.

Doctor: Good. And is your Higher Power taking care of you right now?

Linda: Yes, I believe it is.

Doctor: Is it taking care of the people you love? *(With all of these questions, the doctor is assessing whether or not Linda's spiritual beliefs are positive ones; that is, will her spiritual beliefs aid her in a positive way? Please Note: Obviously, some of your patients will not have a belief system that will aid them in "combating" the monkey in a productive way. For example, some of your patients may tell you that the God of their understanding does not love them and/or does not care for them. They may perceive God as punishing or angry with them because of their drug use. Or, you may have patients who do not have any type of spiritual beliefs. For these types of patients, it may be useful to use the concept of a "wise self"; that is, "Do you believe that you have a wise part of you, a part that loves you and takes care of you even when you might make bad choices? The part of you that gets you to come to the office to reach out for help? The part of you that wants peace and love and joy—just to be happy?" Most patients will answer affirmatively to this question. For your patients who do not* *have either spiritual beliefs or a belief in the wise self [we all have one or two!] ask them to "believe that I believe you have a wise self." These are extremely difficult patients to treat, but they can be helped. It just might take a much longer period of time to be able to connect with them.)*

Linda: Definitely.

Doctor: Excellent! Now let me ask you this: Linda, what is your biggest concern, your biggest worry, right now?

Linda: (immediately beginning to cry) That I will never be happy.

Doctor: (leaning forward close to her) Linda, if your loving, caring Higher Power could talk to you right now, and you and I could hear it, what would it say to you right now to comfort you about your fear that you will never be happy? *(CBT: teaching cognitive restructuring using spiritual beliefs. If Linda did not have any spiritual beliefs—or if her belief was in a punishing, angry Higher Power—but she did acknowledge the presence of a wise self, you might ask instead, "What would your wise self tell you right now to comfort you about your fear that you will never be happy?")*

Linda: (after a pause, sniffling) I guess it would say that everything will be okay.

Doctor: So your Higher Power would tell you that everything will be okay and that you will be happy?

Linda: (nodding) Yes. I think it would tell me that I will be happy. Not to worry. It will all happen the way it is meant to.

Doctor: Yes. Sounds like you do have a very loving Higher Power that really does care about you. I have found that our Higher Power part always says the opposite of our monkey part. So, your Higher Power is telling you, "Everything will be okay. I will be happy. Don't worry. Everything will unfold the way it is meant to." However, your *monkey* is saying, "Everything will *not* be okay," "You'll *never* be happy!" "You better worry because it's all going to be bad!" "Everything is random and you have no control whatsoever!" Am I right?

Linda: (nods and smiles broadly) Exactly. Boy, my monkey really does a number on me, doesn't it?

Doctor: Yes, monkeys are not nice! They do a number on all of us. We talked about your boyfriend earlier. What would your Higher Power tell you about the breakup that would make you feel less upset?" *(Note that the doctor increases rapport by letting her know he has not forgotten about her pain regarding her recent breakup with her boyfriend. If you tell your patient you will "get back" to something she has said, make sure you do—even if you have to write a quick note in the chart to jog your memory before the visit ends.)*

Linda: The same kinds of things. Everything will be okay and I am better off without him right now.

Doctor: Good! It sounds like you have a very strong connection with your Higher Power. You seem to be able to really get in touch with what it says to you. And when you listen to it, you seem to feel less fearful, is that right?

Linda: Yes. I feel more peaceful when I am trying to get in touch with my Higher Power. But it is so hard to do!

Doctor: Yes, it is. The monkey, or fear, really distracts us, doesn't it? I am someone who believes that there are really only two emotions: love and fear. Fear is the monkey. Out of fear springs all of the other uncomfortable feelings: anger, depression, guilt, shame, remorse, regret. So, underneath anger is fear, underneath guilt is fear, and so on.

And then there is the other feeling, which is love—the part of you that is so connected with your Higher Power. Out of love springs joy, peace, happiness, self-acceptance, and so on. So, underneath joy is love, underneath self-acceptance is love. Does all of this make sense so far?

Linda: Yes, very much so. I think I have been listening to my fear a lot.

Doctor: Most of us do. The monkey is *very* loud and gets right in our face and shouts at us! It's hard not to listen to it in the moment. However, once we learn to change our thoughts—to move away from fear and move toward love—we are more able to control how we feel in a given moment. That said, we might *not* be able to change our initial *reactions* to things. I don't think that I will ever become so highly evolved that I won't get upset when somebody cuts me off in traffic! However, I can now control *how long I stay upset*, which is a huge deal.

Linda: Yes, that is what I want to be able to do, too.

Doctor: And you will! So, in addition to following our agreement to stay at the dosage you are on now and to discuss slowly decreasing the Xanax over time at our next visit, here is what I would like to suggest (takes out a prescription pad and writes down the following underlined thoughts):

First, I would like to suggest that you simply <u>become aware of the monkey</u>. The only way we can change, or control, something is to first become aware of it. The way you do this is, anytime you feel anything on the "fear" side, angry, depressed, scared, and so on, stop yourself and simply become aware of what thoughts are creating those feelings. In other words, become aware of the monkey talk.

Second, <u>make a decision to change monkey talk to Higher Power talk.</u> You do this in the same way you did here. Ask yourself, "What would my Higher Power say to me right now to comfort me?" Sometimes we make the decision to continue listening to our monkey. For example, when we get into an argument with a loved one, sometimes we *want* to continue feeling angry or self-righteous. There isn't anything wrong with that, it's simply a very human choice we are making in the moment. However, if you *don't* want to continue to feel distressed, then ask your Higher Power what it would tell you and try to replace the monkey talk with Higher Power talk. I should note that this sounds simple, and, in theory, it is. But it is *not* easy! This exercise can be extremely difficult to do, but it does get easier with practice. One thing you can try to help make this replacing, or restructuring, of thoughts easier is to attempt to do it only when you are feeling *a little* angry, sad, anxious, and so forth. When we are learning something like this, it's good to try it when our emotions aren't really big or extreme because it's hard to learn this when the monkey is shouting at us! However, later on, after you have mastered this technique, you *can* use it to successfully decrease distressful emotions by changing your thoughts—even when the monkey is loud and you are feeling *really* angry, sad, scared, and so forth.

The third thing I would like to suggest is to <u>focus on one day at a time.</u> If you find yourself thinking about the "what ifs" in the future, or the "woulda, coulda, shouldas" of the past, ask yourself, "Is there anything I can do about it today?" If there is, do it! However, if there isn't, bring yourself back to the moment and "let go, let the Higher Power." Trust that everything will work out the way it is meant to, as you said earlier.

By the way, I will be teaching you a technique at our next visit to use to bring you more into the moment and to help keep you out of the future and the past.

So, these are the three things I would suggest that you do before our next visit. Linda, even if you *don't* do the homework, still come back for the visit, okay? Sometimes we get the most information when patients *don't* do the homework. We can find out what is blocking them from doing good things for themselves. Also, just the willingness to *try* to do the homework is healing in itself—the benefits that you actually get from doing the homework are like the icing on the cake!

So Linda, how has all of this been for you, and how are you feeling right now?

Linda: Well, everything you said makes a lot of sense. As I said earlier, my monkey has been really talking to me. I hope I am able to use what you've taught me. I do feel better than I did when I came in today.

Doctor: When you just said, "I hope that I am able to use what you've taught me," I'll bet your monkey was saying, "you won't be able to use any of this" or "you won't be able to do this right!"

Linda: (laughing) I think you know my monkey really well!

Doctor: Yep. As I said earlier, I have a monkey too, and all of our monkeys basically say the same kinds of things to each of us. So, I'll see you in about three weeks so we can check in about how your medication use is going and for another stress management visit. Call the office in the meantime if you need to. Is that okay with you?

Linda: Yes. Thank you, doctor. I'll work on pushing my monkey away—getting it off my back! (smiling)—in the meantime!

Visit Two: From Monkeys to Mindfulness

Linda has returned for her follow-up stress management visit three weeks later.

Doctor: Hi, Linda. How are you?

Linda: (hesitates) Oh, pretty good, I guess.

Doctor: You sound a little unsure. How have you been feeling?

Linda: I guess I have been feeling a little scared. I am still not happy about the idea of cutting down on the Xanax. I've been anxious.

Doctor: Well, it can be scary to think about cutting down on a medication that you have been on so long. Do you remember what we discussed last visit about how this medication works in your system? We talked about this right before we made our agreement *(The doctor is empathic and caring while he is also checking the patient's understanding, as well as trying to see where she is in regard to their previous agreement.)*

Linda: (nods) Yes. You said that this medication will make my anxiety worse if I continue to stay on it. I have been following your advice because, after I thought about it, I guess I don't want to be "addicted" to a medication forever. I probably would be more at peace if I were able to stop taking Xanax, but I am afraid to totally stop it because I am afraid I won't be able to deal with anything. So I really don't think we should go lower than the dosage you gave me last time. *(Note that Linda has now moved to the Contemplation stage of change, which is best seen by her ambivalence. Her previous denial has softened somewhat in that she is exhibiting some insight into her "addiction" to Xanax. However, she is telling the doctor very clearly that she is afraid of stopping the medication right now and does not want to continue to titrate down in terms of dosage. She is "scared" and, as we know from the first visit, "underneath fear is fear" (i.e., the monkey)! Also note that, as discussed in this book, movement from one stage to the next can take years! That is, most of your Precontemplator patients will not come back in the Contemplative stage on their second visit, as Linda has. However, you will have some who do—these are the patients who may be older and/or who have had more consequences (emotional, legal, relational, etc.) as the result of their alcohol/other drug use. We are using this example to illustrate some of the strategies that can be used with your Contemplator patients.)*

Doctor: Linda, I am hearing you say that you do not want to continue with our agreement of slowly taking you off the Xanax while starting you on other, nonaddictive medications.

Linda: (nods)

Doctor: Linda, you said a moment ago that you didn't want to be addicted to Xanax and you thought that you would "probably be more peaceful," but you are afraid to stop it because you think you won't be able to deal with anything—is this right? *(MI: strategies for Contemplators—the doctor is gently pointing out the discrepancy evident in Linda's thoughts.)*

Linda: (softly) Yes.

Doctor: It's normal to feel pulled in two directions when thinking about the pros and cons of making a change. *(MI: strategy for Contemplators—the doctor is normalizing her ambivalence. The doctor may want to use Botelho's Decision Balance chart shown in Figure 5.2.)*

Let me ask you this: What kind of "talk" is the thought, "I would probably be more peaceful if I stopped the Xanax"? Monkey talk or "Higher Power" talk? *(CBT: The doctor is bringing up a topic from the last session and is asking the patient to become of aware again of how her thoughts create her feelings.)*

Linda: Oh, Higher Power talk, for sure. But I am so worried about not being able to cope.

Doctor: Anything after "but" is the monkey! You know, I had given you some "homework" last time we met: to become aware of your negative self-talk, or "the monkey," to make a decision to change thoughts from monkey talk to Higher Power talk, to work on taking things one day at a time. How was that for you? *(Note that the doctor has moved from asking Linda to become aware of her thoughts to discussing and reviewing these concepts further—and to streamline the session by asking about her perceived success or failure with the assigned homework. Remember to always follow up on the homework assigned in the previous visit! Otherwise, the patient may feel that you do not care or that these concepts really are not that important. What is important to you will be important to your patients!)*

Linda: (nods) It was good. I mean, I was able to see how my monkey screws things up for me. It was hard hearing Higher Power talk, as you said it would be, when the Monkey was loud. But, I *was* able to do it a few times.

Doctor: And, during those times when you were able to do it, did you feel a little better?

Linda: Yeah. I felt like there might be some hope.

Doctor: So, Higher Power talk makes you feel hopeful. And you said a moment ago that the knowledge that you would have more peace if you stopped the Xanax came from your Higher Power talk. *(Note that the doctor repeats this positive statement several times.)* What would your Higher Power say *right now* (if I could hear him and you could hear him) to comfort you about your fear that you won't be able to cope or deal with anything if you stopped the Xanax? *(CBT: cognitive restructuring.)*

Linda: (silent for a moment) He would say, "It's going to be okay. Everything will be okay."

Doctor: Good! Linda, I know you are having difficulty believing this Higher Power talk right now and that's okay. Remember, monkey talk is very convincing—even though it's not true! It will take time, but you are definitely on the right path. Have you ever done something positive for yourself that, at the time, you didn't think you would be able to do? *(MI: strategies for Contemplators—elicit ideas regarding the patient's perceived self-efficacy and expectations.)*

Linda: Yes. I got out of a really bad relationship years ago when I didn't think I would ever leave him.

Doctor: Were you afraid at that time that if you left him you might not be able to cope?

Linda: Yes. I thought I wouldn't be able to do anything without him and that I would fall apart and be alone forever if I broke it off. *(Linda's monkey talk is very apparent here. Note that she was probably feeling pretty hopeless after that breakup. She used the term "forever." Terms such as "always," "never," and "forever" are "absolutist" in nature and usually create strong, negative feelings.)*

Doctor: So, the monkey was *really* loud! So, *did* you "fall apart"? Were you unable to do anything without him? *(CBT: confronting "truth" of distorted thinking—what's the evidence?)*

Linda: No. It was actually the opposite. Yeah, at first, it hurt. But I felt a lot better. He really was not good for me. My boyfriend, well, my *ex-*

boyfriend, because he just broke up with me, is kind of like that old boyfriend. (pauses and appears reflective) So, maybe it's actually a *good* thing he left. (*Note that the patient is coming up with these insights and that the doctor was just a "catalyst" in helping her by asking key questions. If the doctor had told Linda that her ex's—past and recent past—were not good for her, it is doubtful that these insights would have been as powerful for Linda. [A word should be said about "key questions": one of the things H.P. has seen physicians worry about the most is, "Am I missing something?" in regard to patient statements. Do not spend time worrying that, because you are not a psychologist or psychiatrist, you may not be asking the "right" questions. Instead, just become aware of the thoughts your patient is describing (his or her "monkey") and, over time, you will find that the really important things will keep coming back until you finally get them! Obviously, always assess, and document that you have assessed, suicidal ideation/plan/intent and psychosis with patients who are new, depressed, anxious and/or who have a psychiatric history in addition to a substance use history. See Chapter 3 on Assessment for further information.]*)

Doctor: Very good insight! Sometimes the things that we think are the worst turn out to be the best. You know, as you were talking, I saw some similarity between what you said about your old boyfriend and what you've said about the Xanax.

Linda: (surprised) Huh?

Doctor: Yes. When you were talking about your old boyfriend, you said that the monkey was telling you that if you left him or "stopped" the relationship, you wouldn't be able to cope and you'd fall apart. The monkey is telling you kind of the same thing will happen if you "leave" your "relationship" with the Xanax. (*Note that you do not need to be a psychologist or psychiatrist to make these kinds of connections. You just need to observe and to really listen to what the patient's monkey is saying.*)

Linda: Yeah. Hmmm, I guess it is, isn't it?

Doctor: I think so. Remember, the monkey always lies! You were okay after leaving your old boyfriend—even though the monkey told you the opposite, weren't you? Let me ask you this: we know what the pros were when you left your old boyfriend; what would be the pros about stopping the Xanax? (*MI: strategies for Contemplators—eliciting and weighing pros and cons of substance use and change. You may want to use Botelho's Decision Balance chart to assist with this process; see Figure 5.2.*)

Linda: Well, like my Higher Power talk said, I would have more peace. I wouldn't have to worry about getting a refill or about finding the money to pay for it. (Linda is quiet for several seconds) My family would be happy that I was off the pills, and I guess I would feel like a better mother to my kids. I guess I would have a lot more energy too.

Doctor: Lots of very great reasons! So, what are the cons of stopping the Xanax?

Linda: (grimacing) Like I said, or like the monkey is telling me, I feel like I might not be able to cope or handle stress and that my anxiety would get worse. I might yell at my kids more if I wasn't kind of numbed out. I don't know, just things like that.

Doctor: All monkey talk—but also very common thoughts of those who are considering stopping a drug that they have relied on for a long time. Because you were able to leave that bad relationship when you thought you couldn't, do you think that you would be able to stop the Xanax—if you really wanted to? *(MI: strategies for Contemplators—self-efficacy.)*

Linda: Yes, I guess. (Then adding quickly) If I really wanted to, which I don't right now. *(Note that Linda is stating very clearly that although she has some belief in her own self-efficacy in being able to stop the medication, she is unwilling to do so at this time. Pushing her at this point will only increase resistance! However, because Linda appears to be slowly moving forward—as evidenced by her openness to discuss this topic, her willingness to come to the second stress management visit, and her decreased use of Xanax, the doctor decides to continue his relationship with Linda.)*

Doctor: Good. If you do become ready to totally stop one day, what could you say to yourself, or what would your Higher Power tell you, to give you motivation to go through with it? *(MI and CBT: emphasizing Linda's free choice and responsibility and self-motivational statement; cognitive restructuring.)*

Linda: (silent for some time) I can do it. I have done hard things before and was okay afterwards. I will have peace. Everything will work out and be okay.

Doctor: Wow. These are excellent self-motivational statements. Your Higher Power talk side is very strong, Linda! *(MI and CBT: elicit self-motivational statements of intent and commitment from patient; cognitive restructuring.)*

So, here is what I would like to suggest: we continue our agreement but, for the next two to three weeks until I see you again, we'll only decrease your dose a tiny bit from the present dosage. We will come back to discussing our agreement next visit. Does that sound okay to you? *(Note that the way in which this doctor handles Linda's resistance toward continuing the contract may differ from the way you handle this dilemma in your office. The point that is being made here is that the doctor feels it is safe to only titrate a small amount (see Chapter 4 for general titration guidelines) because at least Linda will not be taking the high dose she had previously been on and he feels he is moving in the right direction— and he opted for using a strategy for Contemplators [emphasizing the patient's free choice and responsibility for change] rather than utilizing a more heavy-handed approach at this point. The doctor's goal for Linda, however, is still the same: to eventually stop using Xanax. In Chapter 6 we discuss how to handle difficult scenarios such as the "all, nothing, or gray" patients [e.g., those patients at either end of the extreme and those who are stuck somewhere in the middle.] For example, your "all" patient is the one who, after one visit, says that she has completely stopped all her use of the drug and is "doing great!" Your "nothing" patient is the individual who will do nothing in regard to his drug use, takes none of your recommendations, but still comes back expecting you to write him more prescriptions. Your "gray" patient is the one who is stuck in the middle for a very long time without any change; that is, she does not seem to be progressing, nor does she appear to be worsening.)*

Linda: Yes. I can do that.

Doctor: Excellent. Linda, I also want to suggest something else that I think would be very helpful. I would like to recommend that you attend one AA, Alcoholics Anonymous, meeting as an "experiment" over the next couple of weeks. By doing this, you are not saying you have a problem. We, you and I, the "team," if you will, just need to gather some more "data." So, you just go into the meeting and, if you want to, you can sit in the back of the room. You don't have to say anything or interact with anyone at the meeting—even though they are really nice, friendly people—if you do not want to. Basically, this is an experiment to see if you can relate to, or are touched by, anything that is said in the meeting. I have a list of AA meetings in town and would suggest that you attend an open meeting—anyone can attend an open meeting of AA. Closed meetings, however, are just for people who identify that they have a problem. I see you frowning. What are you thinking right now? *(Note that the doctor has taken a risk in recommending to Linda that she go to an AA meeting. Specifically, because he knows that Linda is a Contemplator, the risk is that she may withdraw back into her resistance and shut down. She may feel that the doctor is trying to get her to admit that she has a problem and she may become defensive or angered by this suggestion. However, suggesting trials, such as attending one AA meeting as an "experiment" with no strings attached or judgments made, can be a very useful suggestion for patients in the Contemplative stage. Just be ready for the possibility of resistance!)*

Linda: I am thinking that I don't want to go because I don't really think I have a problem!

Doctor: I know that, Linda. If you find you don't have a problem, then you will never need to go to another AA meeting again and that's okay. What I am suggesting is what I suggest to all of my patients who want to get off a medication but are afraid that they won't be able to cope. If you don't get anything else from the AA meeting, they do talk about a lot of good ways to cope. You don't have to be an alcoholic or an addict to benefit from that, right? *(Note that the doctor does not react to Linda's expected defensiveness with anger or frustration [although it is very easy, and normal, for physicians to feel quite frustrated with patients like Linda!]. Quite the opposite: He joins with Linda by letting her know that if she doesn't have a problem, she'll never need to attend another AA meeting again and that's okay [statement without judgment]. He also normalizes the suggestion ["I suggest this to all of my patients"] and points to the positive outcome of attending an AA meeting [gain insight into new coping strategies] even if she doesn't get anything else from attending the meeting.)*

Linda: (silent for a moment) Well, yes. Okay. I guess I can go to one meeting.

Doctor: That's great! I am really impressed with your willingness, Linda. Your Higher Power talk side is very strong! *(Note that the doctor is* *positively reinforcing Linda's choice. Use positive reinforcement when you want a behavior to continue and/or to increase in frequency.)*

Okay. Now I would like to teach you something that will help you to change thoughts to change feelings. It's called "the awareness exercise." *(Note that the doctor is changing the focus of the visit now that they have come to an agreement. He is now preparing to teach Linda the second nonpharmacologic treatment modality: mindfulness.)*

Have you ever wondered why little children seem so happy? Of course, they also feel lots of other emotions too—anger, sadness, fear— but have you noticed how they seem to keep coming back to a base of happiness? The reason for this may be that they don't have a monkey yet! I mean, how many five year olds do you see worrying about what is going to happen in kindergarten a week from now? Or feeling guilty because of taking their friend's toy three days ago? Little kids rarely, if ever, think about the future or the past. They're so plugged into the moment that their emotions may shift rapidly. For example, a little girl who sees a bird may shriek, "Mommy! Look at the birdie!" and she feels excited. Then, a split second later, "Mommy, will the birdie bite me?" She now feels fearful, and then, another moment later, 'Oh, Mommy, I want to hold the birdie *now*!" And she whines and scowls and feels angry that she can't have what she wants exactly when she wants it. Then, suddenly, another bird flies up to join the first, and she feels happy and excited again.

Linda: (laughs and nods in recognition) Oh, man, I remember when my kids were that little and so in touch with only what was going on in front of their faces. I remember it was so hard to keep up with them— I was still feeling upset and they were already two emotions ahead of me!

Doctor: That's right! The thing is, you and I still have a part of us that remembers when we used to think like that, when we were small kids and only existed in the moment. Remember how long summer used to seem? And now don't those months just seem to fly by? The reason is that when we were kids, we only existed in the present, and time lasted forever because we were so aware of everything around us, minute by minute. Now, as adults, we hardly *ever* stay in the moment—we are so busy planning, worrying, or thinking about the past—and so time moves very quickly. Happiness exists only in the moment. What I am going to do right now is to demonstrate the awareness exercise. I would like for you to just watch me for a few seconds and, when I am finished, to tell me what you saw me doing. There are no wrong answers, and this is not a test. Is that okay?

Linda: (smiles) Sure.

Doctor: Okay, I'll begin. *(The doctor starts to slowly scan the room and take note of the colors he sees, the sounds he hears, and the sensations he feels in the moment. Several seconds go by between each observation.)* I am aware of the silver and brown . . . the red . . . I hear a hum . . . I am aware of the dark and the light . . . my fingertips feel warm . . . the chair is soft . . . I hear someone talking outside the room . . . I see the green and the white. . . . *(The Doctor stops and turns his attention back to Linda, who is listening attentively.)* So, what did you see me do?

Linda: Um, you were aware of the things around you?

Doctor: Good! And what senses did I use to become aware of the things around me?

Linda: Your sight, hearing, touch.

Doctor: Very good! Now, what did you see me *not* doing?

Linda: Um, thinking?

Doctor: Yes! I wasn't "up in my head," thinking. I was simply trying to be aware of the things I saw, heard, and felt. I didn't use smell or taste because I can't really smell or taste anything specific right now. As you said, I wasn't thinking. I had a little break from my monkey and it felt good! Did you notice how I started to slow down a bit?

Linda: Yes.

Doctor: I have been doing this for years, and now it is like my body is "trained" to relax and slow down when I start doing the awareness exercise. Related to not thinking, I also was not judging. Notice that I didn't say, "I am aware of the light on the ceiling . . . and the darkness of the area that is not touched by the light . . . And, speaking of the light—wow! They haven't cleaned up there in a long time and, hey, are those halogen bulbs?"

Linda: (laughs) You didn't *analyze.*

Doctor: Right again! Yes, I didn't analyze or judge. I didn't get stuck in the "paralysis of analysis" that the monkey loves so much. It seems that the more we think, the worse we feel! So, this is a way to think again like a small child, to have the freedom and happiness that young kids have. Another important thing: This is a great strategy to use when we need to "disconnect" from the monkey. By using the awareness exercise to get out of our heads—where the Monkey lives—and to ground ourselves in the moment, we have a chance to change our thoughts to change our feelings. So, in effect, it is a good thing to "lose your mind" in this case! Changing thoughts and feelings is hard to do when we are in our heads, or our "minds," because that monkey is so darn loud!

Linda: Makes sense.

Doctor: Yes, it does. Here's what I would like to suggest: go ahead and continue to be aware of the monkey and continue to work on changing monkey talk to Higher Power talk, as well as focusing on one day at a time. I would also like to suggest that you try to do the awareness exercise three times a day. Do it only for several seconds, and do it when you are *not* feeling especially distressed. Remember, as we discussed at our last visit, when we are trying to learn something, it is best to do it when we are feeling pretty good and *not* when we are feeling really angry, sad, depressed, and so on. The goal, after learning this, *will* be to use it during those difficult times, but it is hard to learn when we are upset. Okay?

Linda: Okay. Should I do it out loud, like you did?

Doctor: Glad you mentioned that. Yes, it is probably best to do it out loud instead of to think it, because, remember, we are trying to get you away from your thoughts (monkey territory). Just don't do it when you are in the waiting room or when you are in a crowded elevator, okay? (smiling)

Linda: (laughing) Okay. I'll try this and the other stuff from last time. And so I am going to be on a lower dose?

Doctor: Yes. Just a little bit lower as I said. You have also agreed today to go to one AA meeting as an experiment and to report back your findings, right?

Linda: Yeah. I'm not crazy about that one, because I really don't feel like I belong there. But, I'll go.

Doctor: Great. Finally, I would like to suggest that you repeat self-motivational statements—"I can do it." "I have done hard things before and was okay afterward." "I will have peace." "Everything will work out and be okay"—every morning when you get up and every night before you go to bed, even though I know you are not ready to totally stop taking the Xanax at this moment. Okay? *(The doctor has written Linda's homework down on a notepad and it looks like this: 1. Continue to be aware of the monkey; continue to make a decision to change monkey talk to Higher Power talk; continue to focus on one day at a time. 2. Awareness exercise three times a day. 3. Attend at least one AA meeting. 4. Every morning and every night, repeat statements: "I can do it." "I have done hard things before and was okay afterwards." "I will have peace." "Everything will work out and be okay.")*

Linda: Okay. Thank you, doctor.

Doctor: Good to see you, Linda. I'll see you back in about three weeks, okay?

Linda: Okay!

Visit Three: Another Way to Stop Monkeying Around—Teaching Your Patient Breathing and Relaxation Exercises

Linda has returned for her follow-up visit three weeks later.

Doctor: Hi, Linda. How are you doing?

Linda: Good. I went to the AA meeting and it wasn't as bad as I had thought.

Doctor: Great! What *did* you think about it?

Linda: Well, they said some good things. And there was this woman who was talking about her addiction to Xanax and I kind of related to a few things that she said.

Doctor: Such as?

Linda: Well, she said that right before she stopped taking the Xanax, she felt really torn.

Doctor: And that's how you feel right now?

Linda: Yes. I do feel that way.

Doctor: Remember what we talked about last time we saw each other, that it is common to feel pulled between two things: whether to continue taking the medication or whether to stop it altogether. Which side are you most leaning toward right now?

Linda: (silent)

Doctor: Linda?

Linda: I guess I am leaning more to the wanting to stop side. I do want to stop taking Xanax, and I do want to try another medication. But I'm still scared. *(By this statement, it appears that Linda is considering change and is, therefore, now in the Preparation stage. Again, it would be highly unusual for a patient to move this quickly from Precontemplation to Preparation, but we are using this example in order to illustrate strategies that can be used with patients in the Preparation stage of change.)*

Doctor: What are the things you are most scared of? *(MI: strategies for Preparators—consider and lower barriers to change. The doctor retrieves the Decision Balance chart that he and Linda completed last visit.)*

Linda: The things we talked about last time (she points to the chart in the doctor's hand). You know, that I won't be able to cope and that I'll get stressed out and my anxiety will get worse. And that I might yell at my kids more if I'm not numbed out.

Doctor: Let's take these fears, or monkey talk, one at a time. Let's say that you stop the Xanax and your worst fear comes true—your anxiety increases and you have difficulty coping. (pauses) What would your Higher Power say to you right now about this fear of being more anxious and not being able to cope with anything?

Linda: I don't know! Well (quiet for a moment) I think my Higher Power would say something like they said at the AA meeting, that "this too shall pass" and that I'll be okay.

Doctor: Excellent. That was one of your self-motivational statements, wasn't it? That "everything will be okay."

Linda: (nods)

Doctor: And what would your Higher Power say to you to comfort you about your other fear—that you will yell at your kids more when you stop taking the Xanax?

Linda: (pauses) Well, I guess something similar, like "everything will be okay—it will all work out." Also, "I'll be a better mom, even if I yell, because I am not numbed out anymore."

Doctor: Great! Those statements are so true. Any anxiety you feel after stopping the Xanax *will* pass, as long as you stay off the Xanax. And you might feel overwhelmed or that you can't cope, but everything *is and will* be okay—as long as you stay off the Xanax. And, you may yell at your kids a little more at first, and maybe you won't, but it *will* all work out, and you *definitely will* be a better Mom when you are no longer taking the Xanax. So, those are great statements to write down and read when you are feeling scared about achieving the goal of stopping the Xanax. What else can you *do*, behaviorally, to help with your fear? Can you call a supportive friend, go to an AA meeting, take a walk, things like this? *(MI: strategies for Preparators—clarify the patient's goal and strategies for change. Notice how the doctor has summarized and emphasized the positivity apparent in Linda's self-motivational [Higher Power talk] statements.)*

Linda: Yeah. I can call my friend Louise. She is the one who has always told me that I don't need to be on medication like Xanax. (pauses) I did kind of like the meeting. I guess I could go to one when I am feeling antsy. And, yeah, I could go for a run. I used to jog all the time before I got hooked on these things. I always used to feel better when I exercised.

Doctor: Those are all great ideas, Linda. Between repeating your Higher Power talk and doing the other things, that old monkey doesn't stand a chance! (smiles)

Linda: Oh, man, from your mouth to my Higher Power ears! (smiles back)

Doctor: Last time you were here, I had suggested some homework (briefly looks at note in chart). You were going to go to an AA meeting, which you have done very successfully! Also, we had discussed that you would continue to be aware of the monkey, continue to make a decision to change monkey talk to Higher Power talk, and keep on focusing on one day at a time. You had also agreed to practice the awareness exercise three times a day and to repeat the statements "I can do it." "I have done hard things before and was okay afterwards." "I will have peace." "Everything will work out and be okay" every morning and every night. How did you do with all of that?

Linda: Okay. I have been getting used to knowing when the monkey is talking to me. Like you said, I always feel bad when I am listening to it. I have been able to get in touch with the Higher Power talk more, but it's still hard sometimes. Sometimes I am not able to hear it until the anger or whatever passes. I know you told me this too, so I haven't really worried about it. That little exercise awareness, has helped too. I noticed that the shade of blue paint on the wall in my house isn't as light as I had thought it was! I notice a lot of little things when I do that exercise, things that I never noticed before.

Doctor: Really good! It sounds like you have been doing a great job with changing thoughts to change feelings and with the awareness exercise. What about the statements every morning and every night?

Linda: Well, I *was* doing it for the first few days after I saw you and then, I kind of forgot (looks sheepish). They did help me when I did do them, though.

Doctor: It's okay that you forgot, Linda. Remember what I told you the first time I gave you a homework assignment—sometimes it's when we *don't* do homework that we get the most information! You said it helped you when you repeated the Higher Power talk, self-motivational statements, yet then you stopped. Do you find that you sometimes do this, stop doing something even though it is helping you?

Linda: Yeah, all the time.

Doctor: What are your thoughts about why that is?

Linda: (silent for a moment) Maybe, maybe I don't feel like I deserve to feel good?

Doctor: That could be a reason. Sounds like monkey talk to me. I tell you what, let's become aware of this and any time you feel like you don't "deserve" something I have suggested, or something that happens in your life, will you tell me about it? And, if you ever want to explore this more deeply, I can give you a referral to a really good therapist. Therapy is great. Everyone can benefit from getting to know themselves better.

Linda: Okay. It may be something I will want to do sometime. And I will try to tell you when I feel like I don't deserve something.

Doctor: Great. And one last thing before I teach you the next strategy—breathing and relaxation. I think that when you have been practicing all of these strategies—changing thoughts to change feelings, mindfulness, and what I will be teaching to you today—in addition to stopping the Xanax, you will feel more and more deserving of good things.

Linda: That's what I hope too.

Doctor: Good. We are on the same page. Now, remember your last visit when we talked about how children live in the moment and that is why they are so happy and carefree? *(Note how the doctor is setting up the introduction to breathing by connecting it with what was done at the last visit.)* Well, in addition to the awareness exercise, there is something else that you can do to help you to become more centered in the moment. What I'd like for you to do is put one hand on your chest and the other on your stomach. *(The doctor demonstrates by putting one hand on his chest and the other on his diaphragm.)*

Linda: (observing him, does the same) Is this right?

Doctor: Yes, very good. Now, take a really deep breath, and, while you are breathing in, pay attention to which hand moves more—the one on your chest or the one on your stomach. (pauses) You might have to breathe in and out a couple of times to really feel which hand is moving the most (pauses several seconds to allow Linda to reflect). Which hand is moving the most?

Linda: (pausing, still appearing to be focusing inward) Umm, I think this one (taps her chest with her hand).

Doctor: When we are "stressed," the hand on our chest moves more. When we are relaxed, or not so stressed, the hand on our stomach, or diaphragm, moves more. One of the reasons that kids may feel happier than we do is that they naturally tend to breathe from their diaphragm. This is another thing that we have "forgotten" to do as we grow older—the other thing is how to live in the moment. So, you can actually reduce your overall stress level by taking in 10 deep breaths from your diaphragm (the doctor taps his stomach) three times a day. Also, remember that thoughts create feelings and feelings, in turn, cause physical sensations that then influence our behaviors, or choices. So, the less stressed you are, the better you will feel physically, which will then help you to make good choices. Does that make sense? *(Note again that the doctor has pulled in information from visits 1 and 2. The more you are able to weave past visits into the current visit, the more powerful the learning of these interrelated concepts is for your patient.)*

Linda: Yes, it does.

Doctor: Good. Let me ask you this: Have you ever done a "relaxation exercise" before?

Linda: Well, I have listened to those tapes where they have the ocean playing.

Doctor: Okay, good. That's a form of relaxation, although not the type we will be doing here today. I also won't be "hypnotizing" you or asking you to do anything that may seem "scary" in any way. In fact, if—while we are doing this brief, six to seven minute exercise—you want to stop at any time, you may do so. What I will be doing is very safe and positive, and I believe it will help you a great deal. In a moment, I will ask you to get into a comfortable position and to close your eyes. I will turn away from you—to give you your "space"—and will close my eyes too. I will ask you to "take a deep breath" many times throughout this exercise. Let the breath out whenever you feel comfortable. Finally, there is no right or wrong way to do this, and if you find you have trouble doing this, don't worry! With practice, you will find this exercise becomes easier and easier. Your monkey does *not* like the idea of you feeling better—or of doing anything that might help you to feel better—so you may find that there is a lot of "noise," that is, judgments, negative thoughts, and so on—in your head while we are doing this. If that's the case, just gently try to push your thoughts away and refocus back on my voice. I know I just said a lot. Do you have any questions?

Linda: No. I think I've got it.

Doctor: Good. Remember, there is no right or wrong way to do this so even if you *didn't* "get it," that would still be okay. Linda, do you like warm baths?

Linda: Um, yes, I love them! *(Note that if Linda had said "no" to this question, the doctor would then use another image to lead her through the beginning of the relaxation. So, instead of water, he may have used "warm, gentle sunlight—not too hot" or another soothing image to systematically help relax specific areas of her body.)*

Doctor: Excellent. What about beaches? Do you find that beaches are relaxing places for you?

Linda: Yes, the most peaceful place I could ever imagine would be a beach.

Doctor: Okay. Before I turn away, if you could rate your anxiety right now, where ten is the worst anxiety you have ever felt and one is no anxiety at all, and a five is somewhere in the middle—what would it be?

Linda: Right now? I guess it would be about a seven.

Doctor: Hmm. It must be difficult feeling that much anxiety. *(When patients give you a high rating of anxiety, pain, depression, stress, etc., it is important to reply with an empathic statement, just to let them know that you heard them and you care. Even exemplary physicians sometimes forget to respond to "rating" responses this way.)* It is my belief that, as we continue to work together, that you will have fewer ratings of seven over time. (pauses) Okay, are you ready to begin the exercise?

Linda: (nods)

Doctor: Good. I'm going to go ahead and turn away from you, as we had discussed, to give you your space. (turns away) Linda, go ahead and close your eyes, if that's okay, and get into a comfortable position. I am closing my eyes too. (pauses) Remember, if you want to stop at any time, you may do so. (pauses) If any thoughts or sounds distract you during the next few minutes, just gently refocus your attention onto my voice. (pauses)

Okay, now take a very deep breath . . . from your diaphragm as we discussed . . . and imagine that your feet are in a wonderful, warm tub of water. . . . The water is the perfect temperature, neither too cool nor too warm . . . just perfect. Take another deep breath and imagine that you have just lowered your legs, from your knees down, into this wonderful bath. . . . You feel very safe and warm. . . . Take another deep breath and allow the water to travel all the way up to your waist. . . . It's as if you've lowered your body from your waist down into this wonderful, soothing bath. . . . You feel the warmth against your lower back and you feel yourself becoming very relaxed. Take another deep breath . . . and imagine that you have a warm, soft towel across your shoulders. . . . The weight of the towel is gently pushing your shoulders down toward the floor. . . . As you take another deep breath you imagine you are slowly lying back in the tub. . . . The towel is cushioning your neck and head and you feel very relaxed and safe. . . . You breathe deeply and feel the warmth of the water on your stomach . . . your chest, your back . . . your arms . . . your hands. You feel yourself becoming more still . . . more peaceful inside. . . . You feel yourself quieting. Take another deep breath. . . . Now imagine that you have a warm washcloth over your eyes. . . . The warmth of the washcloth gently soothes your eyelids. . . . Now your jaws part, and there is a little space between the roof of your mouth and your tongue. . . . You feel very, very relaxed. . . .

I'd now like for you to imagine, as you lie in this warm tub, a beautiful beach . . . almost like you are looking at a snapshot. With your eyes closed, you see the clear blue of the sky . . . the fluffy white clouds . . . the sparkling sand. . . . You feel the soft wind as it blows in from the ocean and touches your face. . . . You feel the warmth of the sun as it gently shines down on your shoulders and hair. . . . You feel the soft sand beneath your feet. . . . You hear the sound of the waves as they roll into the shore. . . . You hear the sound of the wind (pauses) the sound of seagulls in the distance. . . . You taste a little bit of the salt from the sea as it is carried in on the ocean breeze. . . . You smell the freshness of the sea and the warm baked smell of the sand. . . . You feel very much a part of all of this. . . . You feel very safe . . . and relaxed . . . and at peace.

Know that at any time . . . you can come back to this beautiful beach . . . just by closing your eyes and breathing deeply. . . . I am now going to slowly count back from five to one. . . . With each number, you become more aware of being back in this room . . . with all of the sounds outside . . . all of your thoughts . . . but you feel very unaffected by everything around you. . . . Nothing can disturb this peace you have inside . . . unless you choose to allow it to. . . .

Five . . . you begin to become more aware of the sounds outside . . . you turn your head from side to side and stretch a little. . . . Four . . . remember that you can go back to the beach and to this wonderful state of relaxation at any time you want. . . . Three. . . . Two . . . and. . . . One . . . very, very slowly, take your time, you can come back into the room and open your eyes . . . feeling more relaxed and peaceful. *(The doctor slowly and quietly turns around to face the patient once again. When Linda opens her eyes, he speaks in a soft voice.)* Linda . . . please rate your level of anxiety right now . . . without thinking about it too much.

Linda: (thinking) It's about a four right now (she says quietly) *(Most patients will rate their distress lower following this exercise. Of course, you will always have the one or two whose distress is always a ten. For patients who do not report a lessening of distress, tell them that, over time, and with practice, they will see a decrease in their overall level of distress. It's also important to remember that even if Linda had only moved down one point, from seven to six, it would be very important for the physician to "make a big deal" about this—any change for the better, no matter how small, is a great thing!)*

Doctor: Before the relaxation exercise you rated your anxiety as a seven and now, a few minutes later, it's a four.

Linda: (nods and looks somewhat surprised)

Doctor: Isn't that amazing? Nothing has changed. Everything is the same in this room and in your life, but your anxiety went down, *not* because of something "external" causing it to do so, but something "internal," inside of *you* caused the anxiety to decrease. Remember, we can only change what is between our ears, and it appears that you did that really well just now! *(Note that the doctor uses CBT principles, as well as his own observation, along with the "biofeedback" about her self-efficacy she received from witnessing her anxiety decrease, to reinforce this positive result.)*

Linda: Yeah. That *is* pretty cool!

Doctor: I'll say! Okay. Let's make a plan. Do you feel you are at the point where you would like to set a date to completely stop the Xanax? *(MI: strategies for Preparators—the doctor is assessing and clarifying the patient's readiness for following through with her goal.)*

Linda: (pauses) Yes. I think I will be able to deal with my anxiety, because "this too shall pass." I believe, well, I am *starting* to believe that I will be able to do this.

Doctor: That is so great. I know you will be able to do it too, Linda, and, as your doctor, I will be here with you every step of the way. So, I'll go ahead and start decreasing the dosage again and, in about 3 weeks, you should be totally "free" from the Xanax.

Linda: Okay. I guess I had better go back to another AA meeting, huh?

Doctor: Other than stopping the Xanax, that is the wisest decision you could ever make. Actually, the easiest part of stopping a drug is the stopping. The hardest part is staying stopped, and that is where AA can really help you. You will receive a lot of support from the people in AA. Are there other people, like your friend Louise whom you mentioned earlier, who you could call to tell them what you have decided to do and to get their support too? *(MI: strategies for Preparators—help the patient enlist support and publicly announce plans for change.)*

Here is what I would also like to suggest. (The doctor pulls out his prescription pad and begins writing) Number one: Continue to be aware of negative self-talk, monkey talk, and make a decision to change it to change the way you are feeling. Number two: Start attending AA regularly, say, *at least* two to three meetings a week *(Note that the doctor is "setting the bar low." Linda could benefit from attending daily AA meetings at this point, but her doctor wants to let her come to that realization, and he knows that even attending meetings two to three times a week is much more than she is doing now and so will be helpful.)* Number three: Practice the awareness exercise and read your self-motivational statements two times a day—morning and at night. Finally, number four: Take ten deep breaths from your diaphragm three times a day and practice the relaxation exercise at least a couple of times a week. Does that sound okay? Do you have any questions?

> **Linda:** No. I feel like I am getting ready to start a new chapter in my life. I am scared, but really hopeful, for the first time, too. I just have to keep pushing the monkey away and replacing it with "I can do this, no matter what the monkey tells me!" (smiles)

> **Doctor:** You *can* do this, and you *will* be able to do this. The monkey always says the opposite, remember? So, of course it is telling you all kinds of scary, negative things. I am so proud of you, Linda! Let's follow your truth, and stop monkeying around! (smiling) One day at a time.

Appendix 2. Sample Informed Consent and Medication Management and Treatment Agreements

Sample of Informed Consent for Medication Treatment

The purpose of this agreement is to protect you, your access to treatment, including prescribed controlled substances, and our ability to treat and prescribe for you.

The long-term use of such medications as opioids (narcotic analgesics), benzodiazepine tranquilizers, barbiturate sedatives, muscle relaxants, and other medicines to treat pain and addiction is controversial because of uncertainty regarding the extent to which they provide long-term benefit. There is also the risk of an addictive disorder developing or of relapse occurring in a person with a prior addiction. The extent of this risk is not certain.

You are advised and encouraged to review this document and the accompanying practice literature thoroughly and to discuss the decision to undertake medication therapy with your personal physician, loved ones, and legal counsel. Do not sign this document until and unless you have given careful consideration to its contents. The (clinic) physicians are available to discuss any issues regarding their practice and the risks of medication therapy with prospective and current patients.

1. I understand that specific information on risks and potential benefits of individual medications are explained elsewhere, and I acknowledge that I have received such explanation.

2. I understand that some of my medications, including opioids, are classified as Controlled Substances and are subject to a variety of legal constraints as to their prescription, use, and distribution.

3. All controlled substances must come from the physicians at (clinic), unless specific authorization is obtained for an exception. (Multiple sources can lead to untoward drug interactions, including the risk of overdose and death, poor coordination of treatment, and/or legal issues.)

a. If you receive any controlled substances in an emergency situation, you must contact this office with the details as soon as possible. Normally that would be the morning of the next business day and is expected to be within, at most, 72 hours of the situation.

4. I understand that all controlled substances must be obtained at the same pharmacy, when possible. Should the need arise to change pharmacies, I will inform (**clinic**). The pharmacy that I have selected is:

Pharmacy Name: _____   Pharmacy Phone: _____

5. I agree to bring the original containers of medications to each office visit. I understand that I may be requested to bring the original container and any remaining medications to the office for unannounced pill counts between scheduled appointments, and I agree to cooperate with such requests.

6. I understand that **IT IS ILLEGAL TO FURNISH CONTROLLED SUBSTANCES PRESCRIBED FOR MY USE TO ANOTHER PERSON,** and **I AGREE TO TAKE STRICT PRECAUTIONS TO PREVENT UNAUTHORIZED ACCESS TO MY MEDICATIONS.**

7. I agree **TO ADHERE STRICTLY TO MEDICAL INSTRUCTIONS AND LAWS** governing the use of medications and **TO REFRAIN FROM THE USE OF ILLEGAL DRUGS, MEDICATIONS OTHER THAN THOSE PRESCRIBED, OR ALCOHOL** while being seen at (**clinic**).

8. I understand that some of my medications, in particular—opioids, are potentially dangerous and that they may lead to sedation, respiratory depression, **and death.**

9. I understand that medications may be hazardous or lethal to an individual who is not tolerant to their effects, especially a child, and I agree to keep them out of reach of such people and pets.

10. I understand that the effects of sedatives, muscle relaxants, and mind-altering medications or chemicals may be dangerously increased when administered to a patient on opioid medications. I agree to inform other physicians as to which medications I am taking and to request that they consult with my doctor regarding the co-administration of medications that may affect alertness or consciousness.

11. I agree to receive prescriptions for OPIOID and sedative medications **ONLY FROM (clinic) physicians** while I remain under their care and to inform other treating physicians regarding the medications I receive for pain management.

12. I understand that medications may be prescribed alone or in combination and that they may be supplemented with other classes of medications, such as stimulants, tranquilizers, muscle relaxants, laxatives, antihistamines, antinausea medications, or antidepressants. I agree to report to my doctor any of these medications that I am currently taking.

13. I understand that medications, including opioids, may cause a variety of side effects, including, but not limited to, nausea, vomiting, constipation, dry mouth, fluid retention, weight gain, weight loss, suppression of the immune system, suppression of thyroid function, suppression of menstrual cycle, suppression of male hormone, itching, and allergic reactions. I will report any adverse side effects to my doctor.

14. I understand that the medications used to treat pain may impair alertness and coordination. I will not be involved in any activity that may be dangerous to me or someone else if I feel drowsy or am not thinking

clearly. I am aware that even if I do not notice it, my reflexes and reaction time might still be slowed. I understand that such activities include but are not limited to: caring for someone who is unable to care for themselves, working in unprotected heights, or operating heavy equipment. I am aware that **IT IS ILLEGAL TO OPERATE A MOTOR VEHICLE WHEN THE ABILITY TO DRIVE IS IMPAIRED** by such medications, and I agree to comply with such prohibition.

15. I understand that pain and addiction specialists distinguish **PHYSICAL DEPENDENCE** and **TOLERANCE** from **ADDICTION. PHYSICAL DEPENDENCE** and **TOLERANCE** are side effects of certain drugs that usually occur in all patients taking the drug. **ADDICTION** is a distinct and specific diagnosable disease that occurs in a small percentage of patients taking potentially addictive medications. **ADDICTION** is characterized by loss of control of the amount of medication taken, use of a medication even if it causes harm, having cravings for a drug, and a decreased quality of life.

16. I am aware that the development of addiction has been reported rarely in medical journals and is much more common in a person who has a family or personal history of addiction. I agree to tell my doctor my complete and honest personal drug history and that of my family to the best of my knowledge.

17. I understand that OPIOIDS are likely to induce **PHYSICAL DEPENDENCE** and that abrupt withdrawal is likely to cause symptoms such as **increased pain, depression, abdominal and muscle cramps, irritability, nausea, vomiting, sweats, chills, and generalized aching.** I am aware that opioid withdrawal can be uncomfortable but is generally NOT life threatening. However, in some individuals with serious medical conditions, severe withdrawal reactions may be **life threatening.**

18. I understand that medications may be safely discontinued when tapered slowly and that even gradual discontinuation may lead to increased sensitivity to pain. I understand that these medications should not be stopped abruptly, as withdrawal will likely develop. However, I understand that if I am not compliant with this agreement and/or with practice rules, that it may be unsafe for my physician to continue prescribing them. In that situation, I understand that I may be referred to local emergency departments or detoxification units for treatment of withdrawal symptoms.

19. I understand that if I am pregnant or become pregnant while taking opioid medications, my child would be physically dependent on the opioids, and withdrawal could be life threatening for a baby. I am aware that the use of opioids is not generally associated with a risk of birth defects. However, birth defects can occur whether or not the mother is on medicines, and there is always the possibility that my child will have a birth defect while I am taking an opioid.

20. I understand that I am likely to become **TOLERANT** to medications, especially opioids, and that I will probably require increasing doses to achieve adequate pain relief.

21. I understand that Opioid Maintenance Therapy is a controversial treatment and that there is significant disagreement regarding the propri-

ety and morality of such treatment. I understand that the doses of medication prescribed are likely to be significantly higher than doses customarily prescribed for short-term pain management and that physicians and medical facilities unaccustomed to this treatment may refuse to continue maintenance therapy.

22. I understand that certain chronic medical or psychiatric conditions, such as insulin-dependent diabetes, inflammatory bowel disease, sleep apnea, epilepsy, depression, and panic disorder, among others, may increase the risk of opioid therapy and complicate the process of opioid withdrawal.

23. I understand that opioid therapy entails clinical, financial, social, and legal risks. Recent experience suggests a **death rate** among chronic pain patients on opioid therapy of **approximately one death per hundred patients per year** from all causes (not necessarily directly attributable to adverse reactions to medication or drug overdose). Patients relying on insurance reimbursement of medication expenses are subject to denial of coverage based on allegations that the treatment is not medically necessary or that it is unconventional (not supported by the scientific medical literature) and experimental. Chronic pain and opioid therapy may lead to family disagreement regarding the propriety or economic value of treatment, possibly resulting in divorce or estrangement from family members. Employers or regulatory authorities may view opioid therapy as a disqualification for certain kinds of work. Pharmacists and other health care workers may stigmatize patients on opioid therapy as addicts. Possession of opioid medications may make patients the target of robbery or police investigation.

24. I understand that **(this clinic)** is subject to monitoring by regulatory authorities. **I waive any privilege of confidentiality regarding records of my medical care and authorize (clinic physicians) to release copies of my medical records to such authorities.**

25. My signature below signifies that I have read each article in this document and agree to abide by its requirements. I understand that **MY FAILURE TO COMPLY WITH ANY OF THESE REQUIREMENTS CAN CONSTITUTE GROUNDS FOR TERMINATION OF THIS TREATMENT and DISCHARGE FROM THIS PRACTICE.**

Patient's Signature:_____   Date: _____

Witness _____   Date: _____
(First Name, Middle Initial, Last Name)

A copy of this document is provided to the patient at the time of signing, and replacement copies may be requested.

(Reprinted with permission from John B. Hunt, MD, and William S. Jacobs Jr., MD, NexStep Integrated Pain Care, Inc., Jacksonville, Florida (copyrighted material; all rights reserved.)

Sample Medication Management Agreement

The purpose of this agreement is to protect you, your access to treatment, including prescribed controlled substances, and our ability to treat and prescribe for you.

The long-term use of such medications as opioids (narcotic analgesics), benzodiazepine tranquilizers, barbiturate sedatives, muscle relaxants, and other medicines to treat pain and addiction is controversial because of uncertainty regarding the extent to which they provide long-term benefit. There is also the risk of an addictive disorder developing or of relapse occurring in a person with a prior addiction. The extent of this risk is not certain.

Because these drugs have potential for abuse or diversion, strict accountability is necessary. For these reasons the following policies are agreed to by you, the patient, as consideration for, and a condition of, the willingness of this practice to consider the initial and/or continued prescription of controlled substances to treat your chronic pain or addiction.

1. I understand that all controlled substances must come from the physicians at (clinic) unless specific authorization is obtained for an exception. (Multiple sources can lead to untoward drug interactions, including the risk of overdose and death, poor coordination of treatment, and/or legal issues.)

a. I understand that if I receive any controlled substances in an emergency situation, I must contact this office with the details as soon as possible. Ideally, I will contact (clinic) on the morning of the next business day but not later than 72 hours after the situation.

2. I will fill my controlled substance prescriptions at the same pharmacy, when possible. Should the need arise to change pharmacies, I will inform (clinic). The pharmacy that I have selected is:

Pharmacy Name: _____   Pharmacy Phone: _____

3. I agree to take my medication as my doctor has instructed and not to alter the way I take my medication without FIRST contacting my doctor.

4. I will inform my doctor of any new medications or medical conditions and of any adverse effects I experience from any of the medications that I take.

5. I understand that the prescribing physician has permission to discuss all diagnostic and treatment details with other health care professionals who are or have been involved in my care, including dispensing pharmacists, for purposes of maintaining safety and accountability.

6. I agree not to share, sell, or otherwise permit others to have access to these medications. If you suspect I am breaking the law, you may inform law enforcement officials, including the Drug Enforcement Administration.

7. I understand that these medications should not be stopped abruptly, as withdrawal will likely develop.

a. I understand that if I am not compliant with this agreement and/or with practice rules, that it may be unsafe for my physician to continue prescribing them. In that situation, I understand that I may be referred to local emergency departments or detoxification units for treatment of withdrawal symptoms.

8. I agree to cooperate with unannounced urine, blood, breath, hair, saliva, or other specimens requested by my physician. I understand that abnormal test results may prompt referral for assessment and/or treatment for addictive disorder. They may also result in discontinuation of prescribing certain medicines or discharge from care by (clinic).

9. I understand that prescriptions and bottles of these medications may be sought by other individuals with chemical dependency and should be closely safeguarded. I will take the highest possible degree of care with my medication and prescription. I will not leave them where others might see or otherwise have access to them.

a. I understand that because these drugs may be hazardous or lethal to an individual who is not tolerant to their effects, especially a child, I must keep them out of reach of such people and pets.
b. (Clinic) suggests they be kept in lock boxes or safes.

10. I will bring original containers of medications to each office visit.

11. I understand that any medical treatment is initially a trial and that continued prescription is contingent on evidence of benefit.

12. I understand that medications may not be replaced if they are lost, get wet, are destroyed, left on an airplane, etc. (If your medication has been stolen, this is a serious matter, and you should report the theft to the police.)

13. I understand that renewals (refills) are contingent on keeping scheduled appointments. I will not phone for prescriptions after-hours or on weekends.

14. I understand that early refills will generally not be given.

a. Prescriptions may be issued early if the physician or patient will be out of town when a refill is due. These prescriptions may contain instructions to the pharmacist that they not be filled prior to the appropriate date.

15. I understand that if responsible legal authorities have questions concerning my treatment, as might occur, for example, if I were obtaining medications at several pharmacies, all confidentiality is waived, and these authorities may be given full access to our records of controlled substances administration.

16. I understand that failure to adhere to these policies may result in cessation of therapy with controlled substance prescribing by this physician or referral for further specialty assessment.

17. The risks and potential benefits of these therapies are explained elsewhere, and I acknowledge that I have received such explanation.

18. I affirm that I have full right and power to sign and be bound by this agreement and that I have read, understand, and accept all of its terms. All questions have been answered.

I request to proceed with treatment.

_____	_____

Physician Signature	Patient Signature/Date

Date _____	_____

Patient Name (Printed)

A copy of this document is provided to the patient at the time of signing, and replacement copies may be requested.

(Reprinted with permission from John B. Hunt, MD, and William S. Jacobs Jr., MD, NexStep Integrated Pain Care, Inc., Jacksonville, Florida (copyrighted material; all rights reserved.)

Sample Clinic/Patient Treatment Agreement

The purpose of this consent is to protect you, your access to treatment, and our ability to treat and prescribe for you.

1. I agree to keep and be on time to all my scheduled appointments. If I need to cancel my appointment, I will do so a minimum of 24 hours before my scheduled appointment.

2. I agree to adhere to the payment policy outlined by this office.

3. I agree to conduct myself in a courteous manner in the doctor's office.

4. I understand that I may bring one (1) adult guest into the treatment room with me. I understand that (clinic) does not have facilities to care for my children while I am seeing the doctor and that I need to make my own arrangements for their care.

5. I agree not to conduct any illegal or disruptive activities in the doctor's office.

6. I understand that treatment for my condition may involve many different approaches, including medications, injections, physical therapy, counseling, self work, psychological assessments, and others. I will cooperate to the best of my ability with the treatment plan recommended by my doctor.

7. I will inform (clinic) of any new medications or medical conditions and of any adverse effects I experience from any of the medications that I take or treatments I receive.

8. I agree that the (clinic) physicians have permission to discuss all diagnostic and treatment details with other health care professionals who are or have been involved in my care, including dispensing pharmacists, for purposes of maintaining safety and accountability.

9. I will cooperate with unannounced urine, blood, breath, hair, saliva, or other specimens that may be requested. I understand that abnormal test

results may prompt referral for assessment and/or treatment for addictive disorder. They may also result in discontinuation of prescribing certain medicines or discharge from care by (clinic).

10. I will bring my original containers of medications to each office visit. I understand that I may be requested to bring the original container and any remaining medications to the office or pharmacy for unannounced pill counts between scheduled appointments, and I agree to cooperate with such requests.

11. I understand that early refills of medications will generally not be given.

12. I understand that if the responsible legal authorities have questions concerning my treatment, as might occur, for example, if I were obtaining medications at several pharmacies, all confidentiality is waived, and these authorities may be given full access to our records of controlled substances administration.

13. I understand that failure to adhere to these policies may result in cessation of therapy by (clinic) and/or referral for further specialty assessment.

14. I affirm that I have full right and power to sign and be bound by this agreement and that I have read, understand, and accept all of its terms. All questions have been answered.

I request to proceed with treatment.

_____

Physician Signature

Date _____

_____

Patient Signature/Date

_____

Patient Name (Printed)

A copy of this document is provided to the patient at the time of signing, and replacement copies may be requested.

(Reprinted with permission from John B. Hunt, MD, and William S. Jacobs Jr., MD, NexStep Integrated Pain Care, Inc., Jacksonville, Florida (copyrighted material; all rights reserved.)

Index